High-Throughput Screening for Drug Discovery

Edited by Shailendra K. Saxena

Published in London, United Kingdom

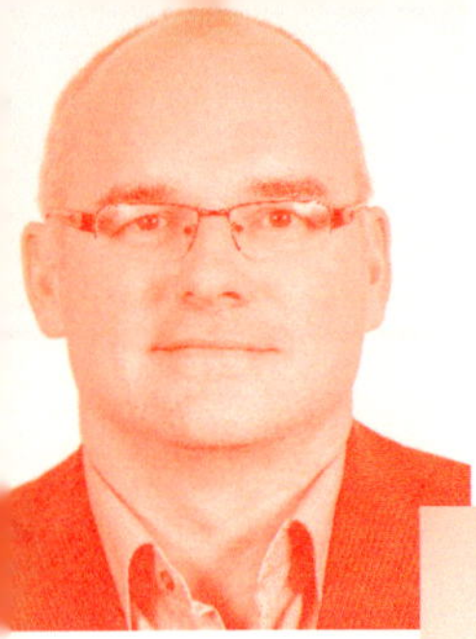
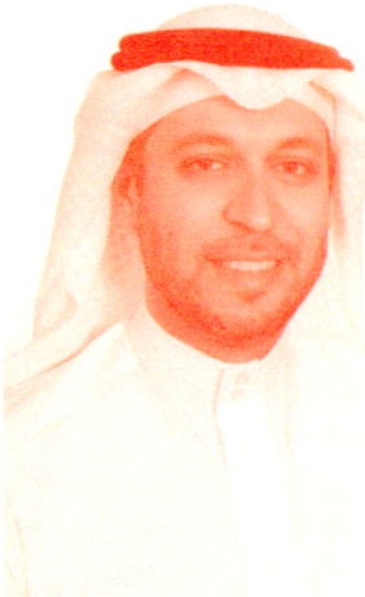
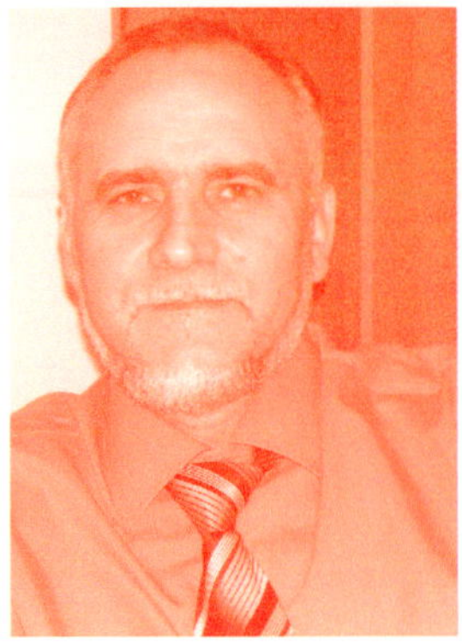
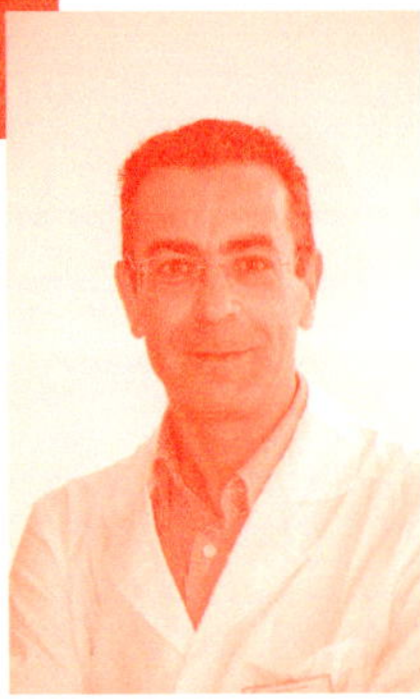
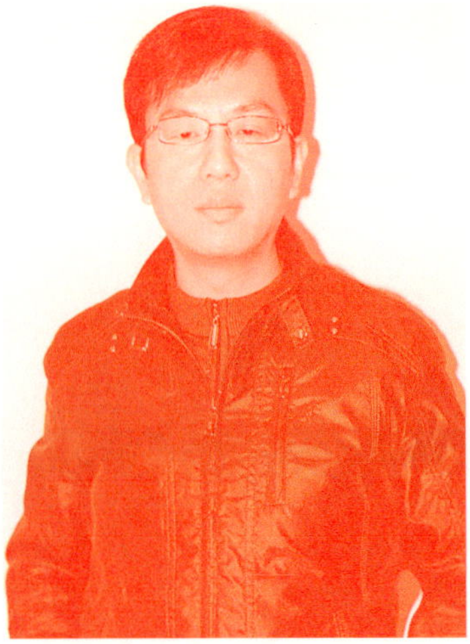
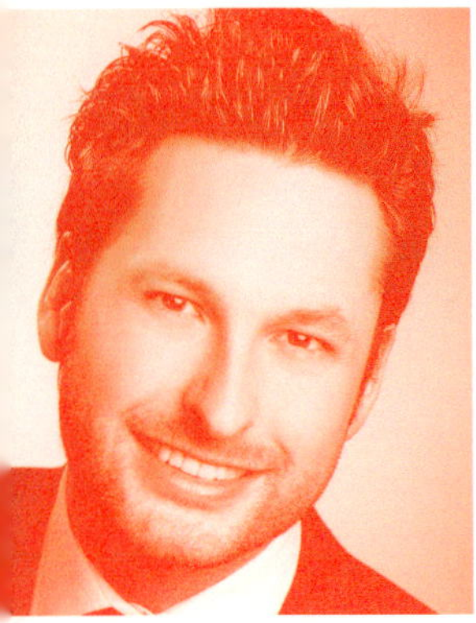
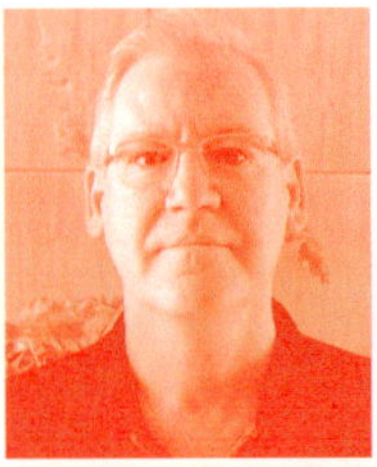

IntechOpen

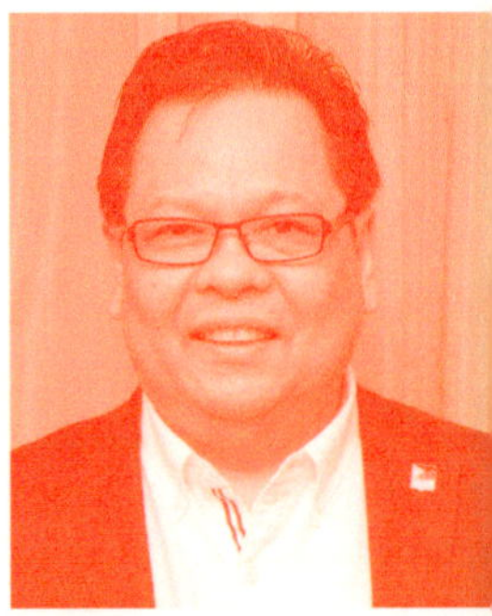
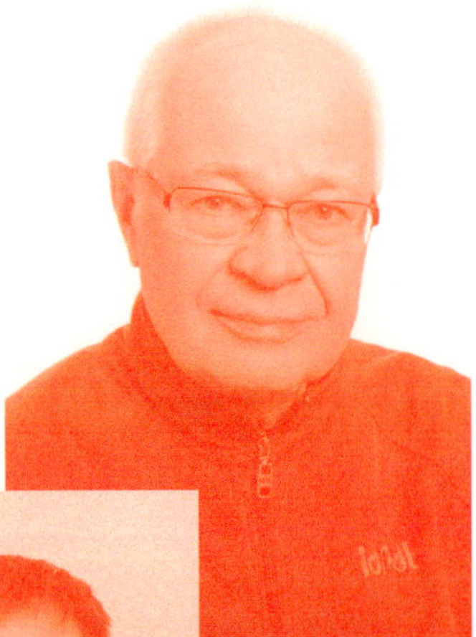
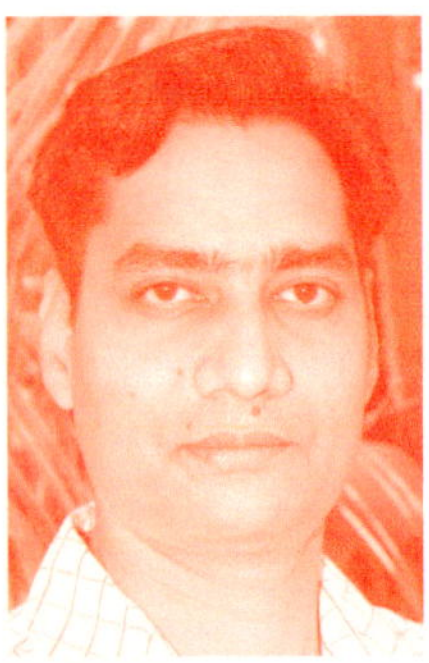
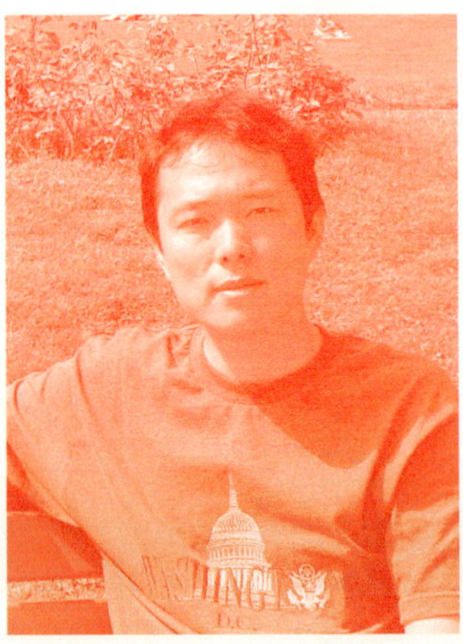
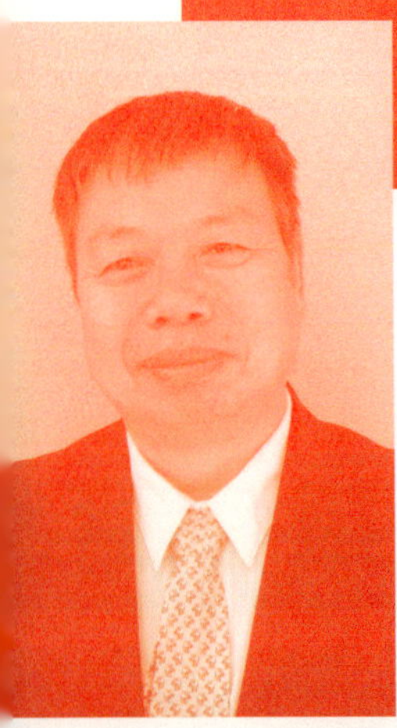
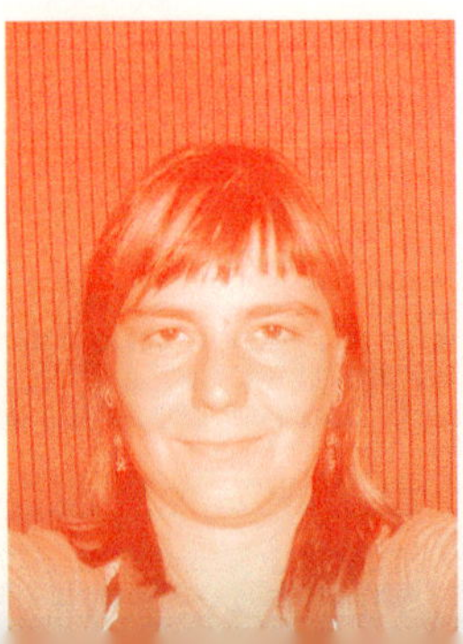

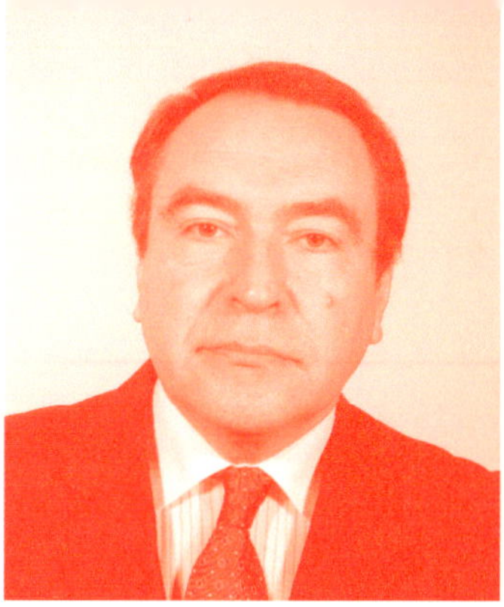

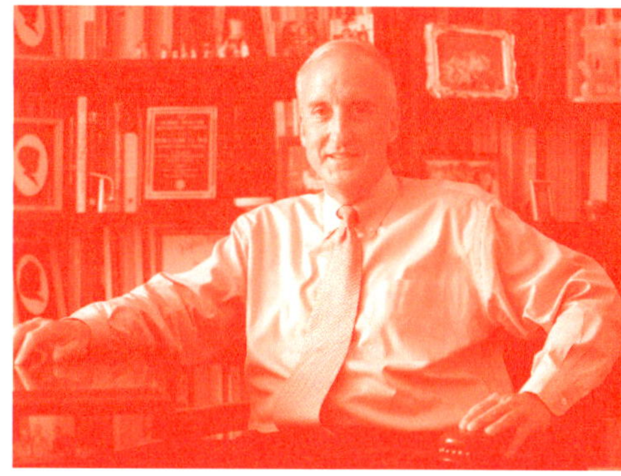

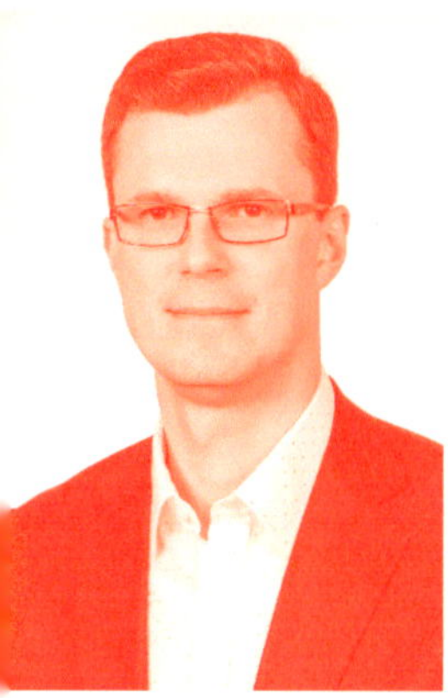

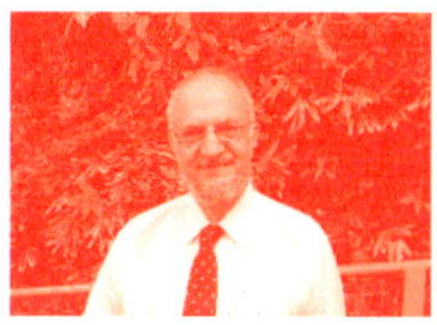

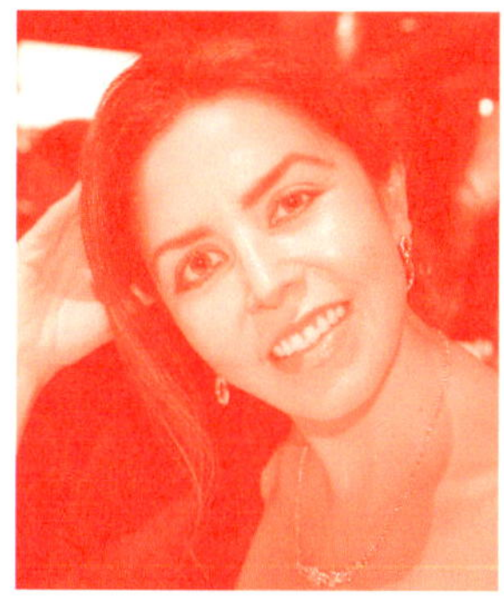

Supporting open minds since 2005

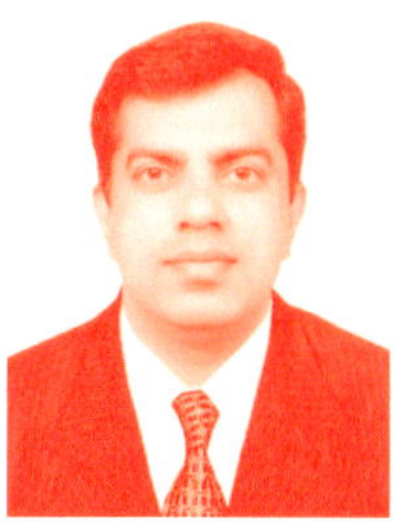

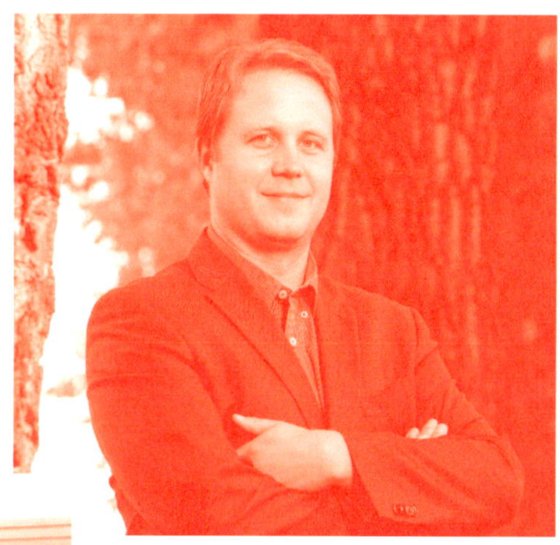

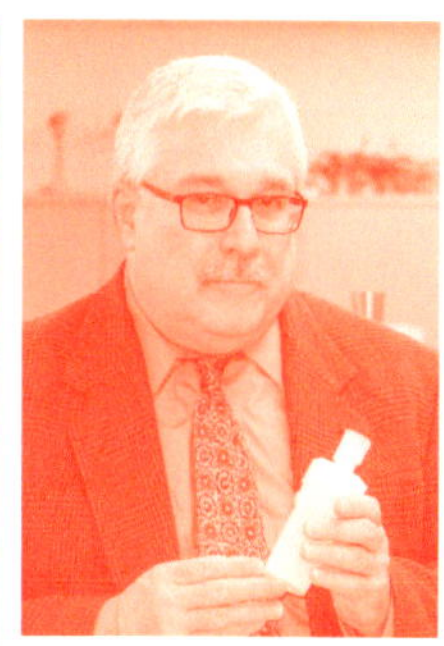

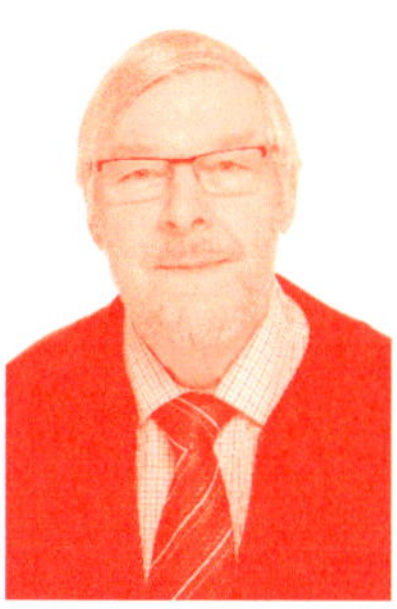

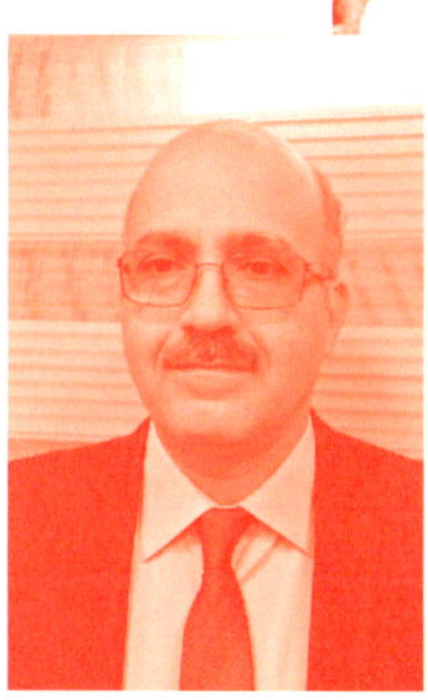

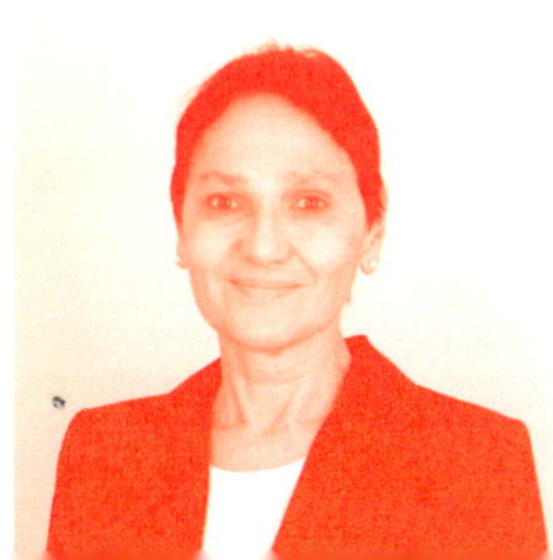

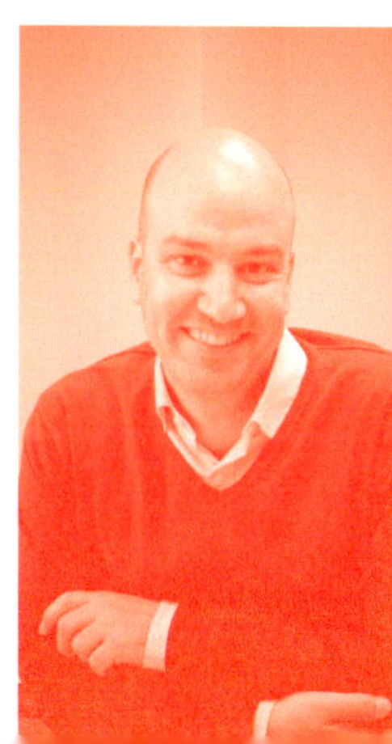

High-Throughput Screening for Drug Discovery
http://dx.doi.org/10.5772/intechopen.91075
Edited by Shailendra K. Saxena

Contributors
Zhaoping Liu, Nina Senutovitch, Andrea Gomez-Donart, Caroline Weldon, John O'Rourke, Nadia Martinez-Martin, Shengya Cao, Fawzi Faisal Bokhari, Ashwag Albukhari, Khaled Hasaan Barakat, Ayman O.S. El-Kadi, Farag E.S. Mosa, Shailendra K. Saxena, Vimal K. Maurya, Saniya Ansari, Swatantra Kumar, Shivani Maurya, Ankur Gupta, Anil K. Tripathi, Bipin Puri

First published in London, United Kingdom, 2022 by IntechOpen
IntechOpen is the global imprint of INTECHOPEN LIMITED, registered in England and Wales, registration number: 11086078, 5 Princes Gate Court, London, SW7 2QJ, United Kingdom
Printed in Croatia

British Library Cataloguing-in-Publication Data
A catalogue record for this book is available from the British Library

Additional hard and PDF copies can be obtained from orders@intechopen.com

High-Throughput Screening for Drug Discovery
Edited by Shailendra K. Saxena
p. cm.
Print ISBN 978-1-83962-947-1
Online ISBN 978-1-83962-948-8
eBook (PDF) ISBN 978-1-83962-949-5

For EU product safety concerns:
IN TECH d.o.o., Prolaz Marije Krucifikse Kozulić 3, 51000 Rijeka, Croatia, info@intechopen.com or visit our website at intechopen.com.

Meet the editor

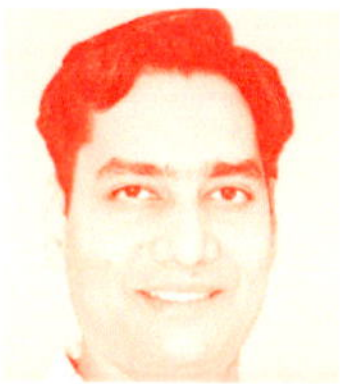

Professor Dr. Shailendra K. Saxena is a vice dean and professor at King George's Medical University, Lucknow, India. His research interests involve understanding the molecular mechanisms of host defense during human viral infections and developing new predictive, preventive, and therapeutic strategies for them using Japanese encephalitis virus (JEV), HIV, and emerging viruses as a model via stem cell and cell culture technologies. His research work has been published in various high-impact factor journals (*Science, PNAS, Nature Medicine*) with a high number of citations. He has received many awards and honors in India and abroad including various Young Scientist Awards, BBSRC India Partnering Award, and Dr. JC Bose National Award of Department of Biotechnology, Min. of Science and Technology, Govt. of India. Dr. Saxena is a fellow of various prestigious international societies/academies including the Royal College of Pathologists, United Kingdom; Royal Society of Medicine, London; Royal Society of Biology, United Kingdom; Royal Society of Chemistry, London; and Academy of Translational Medicine Professionals, Austria. He was named a Global Leader in Science by *The Scientist*. He is also an international opinion leader/expert in vaccination for Japanese encephalitis by IPIC (UK).

Contents

Dedication

Dedicated
to my Parents & Family
who believed in academics
as the way forward for an intelligent mind
and
to the Teachers
who introduced me to the subject
and nurtured my interest in it.

Preface

This book provides a comprehensive overview of high-throughput screening (HTS) and its role in the development of novel drugs for precision medicine, infectious diseases, and cell signaling modulators. It highlights recent advancements as well as future directions in the field. The book focuses on various aspects of HTS for drug discovery for various communicable and non-communicable diseases. HTS is a widely used procedure for identifying bioactive compounds. The function of a target (typically a protein) is determined in presence of a library of compounds for their ability to induce the desired modification. The objective of HTS is to identify the lead compounds that can be developed into drugs of choice. The fact that compound discovery is driven by functional activity rather than known binding is a significant advantage of using HTS. HTS is a well-established method for identifying chemical starting points for drug discovery, with most pharmaceutical companies now screening hundreds of thousands or millions of compounds against a protein of interest. As a result, one of the most valuable assets a pharmaceutical company possesses is its library of HTS-ready compounds. HTS has recently been made possible by advances in robotics, liquid handling, plate reader detection, and high-speed computers. Nonetheless, HTS still necessitates a highly specialized and costly screening facility, which not every lab can afford. Instead of establishing their own facility, institutions with limited budgets typically use HTS services provided by third-party providers such as contract research organizations (CROs) or, more commonly in an academic setting, core facilities.

Using HTS, we can now perform an exhaustive number of measurements in a short period of time using high-throughput technologies, giving access to individuals' DNA (genomics), transcribed RNA from genes over time (transcriptomics), DNA methylation and protein profiles of specific tissues and cells (epigenomics and proteomics), metabolites (metabolomics), and other types of omics data that helps to identify the role of HTS in personalized and precision medicine. This book focuses on the understanding of HTS from various perspectives while discussing the crucial aspect of drug discovery. It is a self-contained collection of scholarly contributions targeting an audience of practicing researchers, academics, Ph.D. students, and other scientists.

I am overwhelmed in all humbleness and gratefulness to acknowledge all the contributors who trusted me and supported me in this work. My research fellows and students are central to all my research and academic work. They are the motivating force behind anything constructive I do. They are truly brilliant and have a bright future. I would like to express gratitude to our mentors, teachers, and students who gave me the strength to see this project to fruition. Also, I would like to thank the colleagues, family, and friends who provided encouragement and support. A happy environment at home is essential for any kind of growth, and I thank my family, especially my talented wife and children, for the same.

Dr. Shailendra K. Saxena
Professor,
Center for Advanced Research (CFAR),
Faculty of Medicine,
King George's Medical University (KGMU),
Lucknow, India

Section 1

Introduction: High-Throughput Screening Based Drug Discovery for Precision Medicine

Chapter 1

Introductory Chapter: High-Throughput Screening - A New Tool for Precision Medicine

Shailendra K. Saxena, Vimal K. Maurya, Saniya Ansari, Swatantra Kumar, Shivani Maurya, Ankur Gupta, Anil K. Tripathi and Bipin Puri

1. Introduction

High-Throughput Screening (HTS) is a programmed process that can rapidly identify active compounds (chemical /biological), antibodies, genes, or one or more candidates based on specific criteria [1]. In the pharmaceutical industry, HTS has been applied for novel drug discovery to overcome the conventional "trial and error" strategies to discover new therapeutic targets or validate their biological effects. Thus, a large number of biological effectors and modulators can be screened against specific targets in a short period using HTS technology during humanitarian emergencies [2]. HTS can also be used to evaluate pharmacological targets and pharmacological profile of agonists and antagonists for various receptors such as G-protein-coupled receptors (GPCRs) and enzymes. In recent years, a large number of drugs in clinical trials have come through HTS campaigns, establishing HTS as a reliable hit-finding technique. HTS has recently emerged as one of the important methods in the area of drug and vaccine design [3–6]. It also allows the immediate incorporation of broad screening collections such as GPCR, kinase, and ion channel-based libraries, as well as the use of client-supplied libraries, into an HTS campaign [7]. Over the past decades, HTS mainly focused on several fundamental technologies like homogeneous assays, high-density microplates, high-performance microliter dispensers, imaging, laboratory automation, and combinatorial chemistry and genomics [8]. The success of HTS is dependent on the identification of meaningful assay systems. HTS is mainly performed using *in silico* methods (ligand-based drug design and structure-based drug design) *in vitro* methods (cell-based assays and biochemical assays), *in-vivo* methods (whole organism-based assays) [9].

Recently, with a rising need to store, access, and compute more sequencing reads and other biological data, HTS technology is becoming more important in the therapeutic context [10]. High-throughput biochemical measures of new variation, thorough health records, and open data sharing will improve our capacity to read individual genomics and understand exactly human health and diseases. The availability of HTS has surpassed current procedures for reporting on data analysis techniques. Lower prices and better accessibility led to an influx of data and related studies, which helped to progress bioinformatics. Innovative, dependable, and accurate omics-based study (i.e., genomics, transcriptomics, and proteomics) would aid novel drug development and precision medicine research [11].

This book also provides an in-depth look at the technologies utilized to detect biological reactions in HTS bioassays, such as fluorescence, luminescence, and atomic absorbance. In the context of anti-infective drug design, discovery, and development, the applications of HTS, reverse pharmacology, present obstacles, and future views of HTS in the pharmaceutical and biotechnology industries are explored. In this book, we describe a novel, multiplex immuno-assay platform based on high-throughput flow cytometry technology and advanced computational algorithms for data analysis. The assay simultaneously measures T cell dynamics including phenotype, time-dependent expression of activation markers, secreted effector cytokines, and proliferation. Further, this book covers the recent advances that use high-throughput methods to move towards the generation of a comprehensive network of extracellular protein-protein interactions (ePPIs) in humans for future targeted drug discovery. Furthermore, the book focuses on the advancement of technologies in HTS methods and research advances in three major technology areas including miniaturization, automation and robotics, and artificial intelligence, which promises to help speed up the discovery of medicines and their development process. At last, this book provides comprehensive knowledge about the use of various machine-learning algorithms for the screening of Aryl hydrocarbon receptor (AhR) modulators that have minimum errors compared with structure-based methods.

Precision medicine has gained a lot of attention in recent years due to its unique approach i.e., "to target the right treatments to the right patients at the right time". According to the National Institutes of Health (NIH), precision medicine is a new therapy and preventative strategy based on knowledge about an individual's genes,

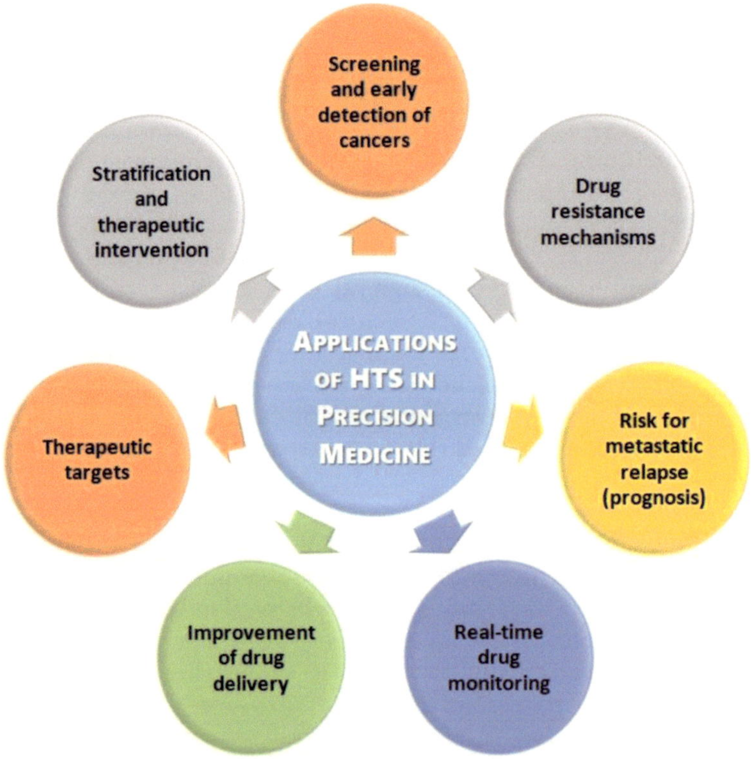

Figure 1.
Applications of precision medicine in cancer management, therapeutic drug monitoring, drug discovery and delivery.

Area	Biomarkers	Treatment	Disease
Infectious diseases	CD4 + T cells, HIV viral load	Highly active antiretroviral therapy	HIV/AIDS
Cancer	BCR-ABL1	Blinatumomab, Bosutinib, Busulfan, Imatinib, Nilotinib	CML
	EML4-ALK	Crizotinib, Brigatinib, Alectinib	Lung cancer
Cardiovascular disease	CYP2C19	Citalopram, Clobazam, Doxepin, Clopidogrel, Carisoprodol	Coronary artery disease (CAD)
Pulmonary disease	G551D	Ivacaftor	Cystic fibrosis
Endocrine disease	RET	Prophylactic thyroidectomy, Carbozantinib	Multiple endocrine neoplasia type 2
Hematology	Factor V Leiden	Avoid prothrombotic drugs	Thrombosis
	Hepatitis C viral load	Direct-acting antiviral agents	Hepatitis C
Metabolic disease	LDL cholesterol	Statins	Hyperlipidemia
Neurology	CXCL13	Immunotherapy	Autoimmune encephalitis
Psychiatry	GRIK1	Topiramate	Alcohol use disorder
Renal disease	Urinary gene signature	Antirejection drugs	Transplant rejection
Ophthalmology	RPE65	Gene therapy	Leber's congenital amaurosis
Pharmacogenomics	CYP2A6	Varenicline	Smoking cessation

Table 1.
Examples of precision medicine applications for the management of various clinical conditions.

environment, and lifestyle [12, 13]. Precision medicine aims to give accurate and personalized treatment to patients by using genomes, proteomics, and other related technologies to evaluate and identify biomarkers in huge sample groups for specific diseases [14]. Precision medicine attempts to limit medical expenses while achieving an optimal treatment impact by bringing humanism, ethics, economics, sociology, and other knowledge factors together [15]. Precision medicine is a new medical concept for gaining a comprehensive knowledge of a patient's genetic and genomic data to estimate disease and make better preventive, diagnostic, and treatment decisions [16]. Medical oncology has progressed through three stages: cytotoxic chemical treatment, gene-driven precision medicine, and personalized molecule-targeted treatment (**Figure 1**) [17]. Precision medicine has entered a new phase in clinical practice today. Its overall purpose is to minimize mortality, morbidity, and disability from serious diseases, improve healthcare service quality (**Table 1**) [18, 19].

2. Applications of high throughput screening (HTS) in precision medicine

Improvements in sequencing technology over the last 10 years have allowed several high-throughput sequencing platforms to provide novel insights to design

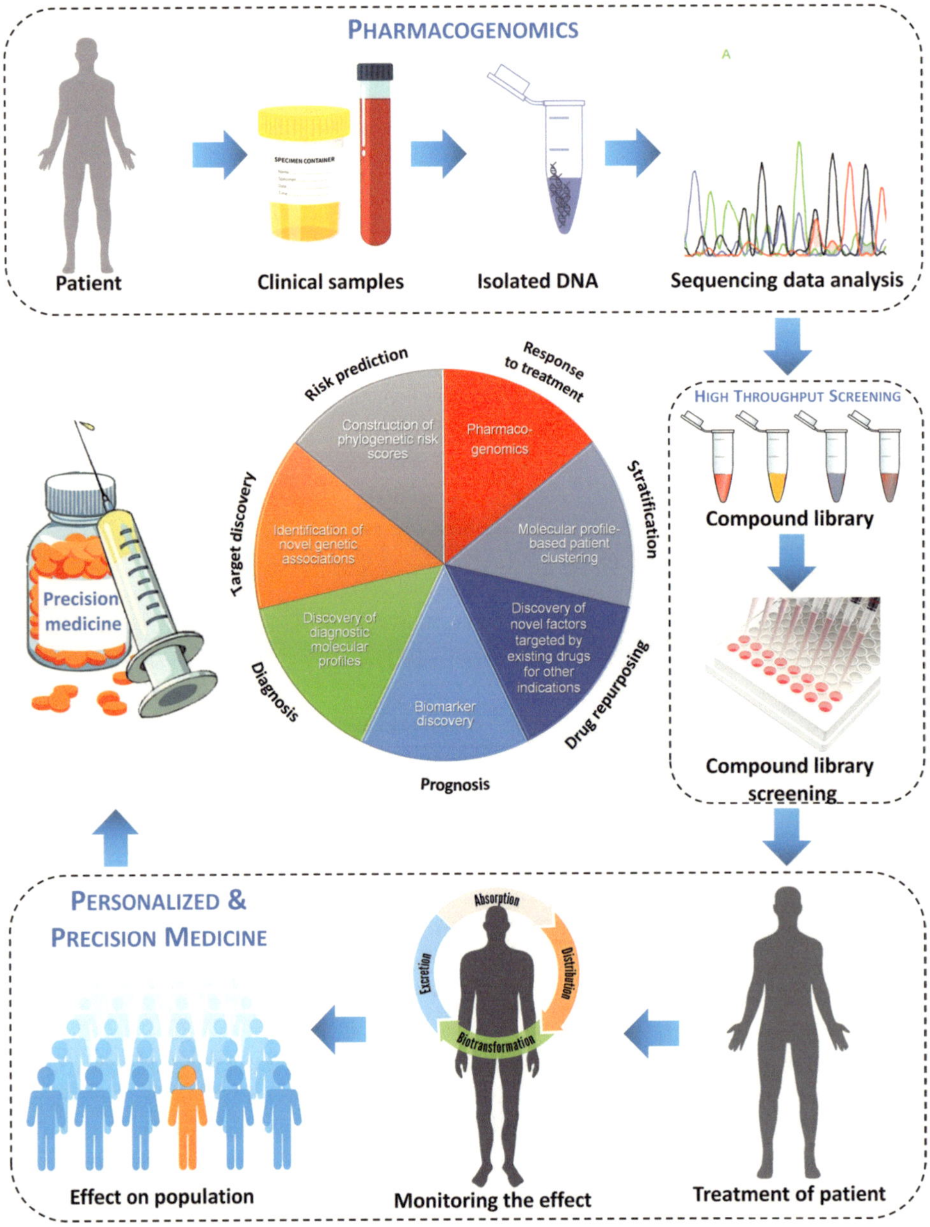

Figure 2.
Scheme for the high-throughput screening based development of personalized/precision medicine. Samples collected from the patients are subjected to DNA isolation and sequencing (NGS) for pharmacogenomics. Based on the analysis of sequencing (NGS) data, high-throughput screening (HTS) of the compound library is performed to identify the drug(s) of choice. Patient treatment with these drug(s) is monitored for its therapeutic and ADME profile. Based on the therapeutic effect of the drug(s), multi-population genome-wide association studies (GWAS) study may lead to development of personalized/precision medicine.

personalized medicine [20]. Modern sequencing technology (Ion, Illumina, Torrent, Oxford Nanopore Technologies, pacific biosciences, etc.) created new paths for HTS in the area of medicine. Epigenetic applications, Genomic (DNA-seq), and transcriptomic (RNA-seq), are all part of HTS. To determine genomic variants (insertion or deletion, single nucleotide variants, copy number alterations, and fundamental changes) from biological samples, whole-genome sequencing (WGS), and whole-exome sequencing (WES) is used (**Figure 2**) [21, 22].

Identification of new transcripts, characterization of gene expression profiles, alternative splicing, RNA editing, and fusion transcripts are all feasible using RNA-seq. [23]. Similarly, next-generation sequencing (NGS) may quickly identify or "sequence" huge parts of a person's genome and are significant advancements in precision medicine clinical applications. These tests can assist patients, doctors, and researchers uncover genetic variations that can help them diagnose, treat, and know more about human disease. Apart from this, NGS techniques can also be applied in the area of metagenomics, RNAseq, ribosome profiling, targeted sequencing, and minor variant reconstruction, as well as a wide range of post-pipeline studies that combine genomic, clinical, epidemiological, and ecological data [24, 25].

HTS has mostly been applied to specific areas of the genome or in the context of identifying microscopic pathogens. Prenatal assays intended to identify chromosomal abnormalities in cell-free DNA from maternal blood are clinically accessible [26]. Targeted HTS of clinically actionable mutations is also being used to guide illness diagnosis and therapy [27]. HTS has also been used in clinical settings to track pathogen outbreaks like methicillin-resistant *Staphylococcus aureus* infections. The development and usage of these specialized assays will continue to grow, but precision medicine depends on the potential therapeutic use of more extensive methods like WGS, which is still facing complications. WGS is the most comprehensive technique for potential therapeutic use since that marks the next stage in the path to a complete understanding of the genetic determinants of a patient's heritable character [28]. Additional genome sequencing, and data from large-scale genomics efforts like ENCODE and GTEx, which allow the development of even more extensive datasets, will help interpret the variations. Community resources for correlating phenotypes to sequences will be provided through open access programs including the Personal Genomes Project and integrated Personal Omics Profiling [29].

3. Few prime areas of high throughput screening (HTS) for precision medicine

3.1 Management of infectious diseases

Efforts have recently been made to combine these technologies with bioinformatics and epidemiology to improve public health surveillance, investigations, and control of infectious diseases [30]. The previous 40 years had a substantial influence on the knowledge of infectious diseases. A broad spectrum of medically important viruses, bacteria, parasites, fungus, and other pathogens have been studied using next-generation sequencing [31]. Many of these pathogens are directly important to the development and assessment of vaccinations, medicines, infection control, and a variety of nonmedical pandemic countermeasures [32].

3.2 Management of cancer

Recently HTS has been coupled with various sequencing techniques in the design of precision medicine for the treatment of various types of cancers like multiple myeloma, glioblastoma, and pediatric cancers. A wide range of FDA approved drugs such as temsirolimus (mTOR inhibitor), ceritinib (ALK inhibitor), and BI2536 (PLK1 inhibitor), panobinostat, bortezomib, ixazomib, carfilzomib, and selinexor, bortezomib (proteasome inhibitor), Bcl-2 inhibitor ABT-263 with the mTOR inhibitor AZD-8055 have been tested as precision therapy for multiple myeloma, glioblastoma, and pediatric cancer [33–35].

4. Conclusions

In clinical and preclinical research, there have been a few attempts to integrate throughput screening technologies with precision medicine. The relevance of high-throughput screening approaches in identifying and designing precision therapies for the treatment of various diseases is highlighted in this chapter. Over the last ten years, advances in sequencing technology have enabled several high-throughput sequencing platforms to bring unique insights into the creation of customized medicine. The sequencing technologies of the present day (Ion, Illumina, Torrent, Oxford Nanopore Technologies, pacific biosciences) created a new roadmap for HTS technologies to identify and design precision therapeutics.

5. Future perspectives

The development of a single definition for precision medicine will aid transdisciplinary areas with a shared understanding of concepts and enhance collaborative ideas. Standardization of HTS and analytical methods will make it easier to validate and replicate findings in clinically relevant timeframes. This, along with interdisciplinary cooperation, will allow it to be fully integrated into patient care and treatment via the development of novel diagnostic, predictive, and prognostic tests. The creation of broad conceptual frameworks that address the underlying drivers of health across specialized areas will be facilitated by the establishment of a shared precision medicine definition, which will promote collaboration between the transdisciplinary domains that make up precision medicine. It may be beneficial to establish a set of recommendations in the next 5–10 years to assist in deciding whether or not research activities or therapies fit precision medicine requirements. These principles might determine if the endeavor should include efforts to personalize therapies, a focus on genetics/biology, the environment, nutrition, and/or lifestyle, as well as the amount to which these distinct variables interact.

Author details

Shailendra K. Saxena[1*], Vimal K. Maurya[1], Saniya Ansari[1], Swatantra Kumar[1], Shivani Maurya[1], Ankur Gupta[2], Anil K. Tripathi[1] and Bipin Puri[1]

1 Centre for Advanced Research (CFAR), Faculty of Medicine, King George's Medical University (KGMU), Lucknow, Uttar Pradesh, India

2 Government Pharmacy College, Sajong, Rumtek, Sikkim, India

*Address all correspondence to: shailen@kgmcindia.edu

References

[1] Szymański P, Markowicz M, Mikiciuk-Olasik E. Adaptation of high-throughput screening in drug discovery-toxicological screening tests. International Journal of Molecular Sciences. 2012;**13**(1):427-452. DOI: 10.3390/ijms13010427

[2] Sachinidis A. High-throughput base editing: A promising technology for precision medicine and drug discovery. Signal Transduction and Targeted Therapy. 2021;**6**(1):221. DOI: 10.1038/s41392-021-00633-0

[3] Maurya VK, Kumar S, Prasad AK, Bhatt MLB, Saxena SK. Structure-based drug designing for potential antiviral activity of selected natural products from Ayurveda against SARS-CoV-2 spike glycoprotein and its cellular receptor. VirusDisease. 2020;**31**(2):179-193. DOI: 10.1007/s13337-020-00598-8

[4] Maurya VK, Kumar S, Bhatt MLB, Saxena SK. Antiviral activity of traditional medicinal plants from Ayurveda against SARS-CoV-2 infection. Journal of Biomolecular Structure and Dynamics. 2022;**40**(4):1719-1735. DOI: 10.1080/07391102.2020.1832577

[5] Mishra S, Maurya VK, Kumar S, Ankita KA, Saxena SK. Clinical management and therapeutic strategies for the thyroid-associated Ophthalmopathy: Current and future perspectives. Current Eye Research. 2020;**45**(11):1325-1341. DOI: 10.1080/02713683.2020.1776331

[6] Kumar S, Maurya VK, Prasad AK, Bhatt MLB, Saxena SK. Structural, glycosylation and antigenic variation between 2019 novel coronavirus (2019-nCoV) and SARS coronavirus (SARS-CoV). VirusDisease. 2020;**31**(1):13-21. DOI: 10.1007/s13337-020-00571-5

[7] Aldewachi H, Al-Zidan RN, Conner MT, Salman MM. High-throughput screening platforms in the discovery of novel drugs for neurodegenerative diseases. Bioengineering (Basel). 2021;**8**(2):30. DOI: 10.3390/bioengineering8020030

[8] Shinn P, Chen L, Ferrer M, et al. High-throughput screening for drug combinations. Methods in Molecular Biology. 2019;**1939**:11-35. DOI: 10.1007/978-1-4939-9089-4_2

[9] Gorshkov K, Chen CZ, Marshall RE, et al. Advancing precision medicine with personalized drug screening. Drug Discovery Today. 2019;**24**(1):272-278. DOI: 10.1016/j.drudis.2018.08.010

[10] Trombetta RP, Dunman PM, Schwarz EM, Kates SL, Awad HA. A high-throughput screening approach to repurpose FDA-approved drugs for bactericidal applications against staphylococcus aureus small-colony variants. mSphere. 2018;**3**(5): e00422-e00418. DOI: 10.1128/mSphere.00422-18

[11] Williams JR, Lorenzo D, Salerno J, Yeh VM, Mitrani VB, Kripalani S. Current applications of precision medicine: A bibliometric analysis. Personalized Medicine. 2019;**16**(4): 351-359. DOI: 10.2217/pme-2018-0089

[12] Manzari MT, Shamay Y, Kiguchi H, Rosen N, Scaltriti M, Heller DA. Targeted drug delivery strategies for precision medicines. Nature Reviews Materials. 2021;**6**(4):351-370. DOI: 10.1038/s41578-020-00269-6

[13] Collins H, Calvo S, Greenberg K, Forman Neall L, Morrison S. Information needs in the precision medicine era: How genetics home reference can help. Interactive Journal of Medical Research. 2016;**5**(2):e13. DOI: 10.2196/ijmr.5199

[14] Lightbody G, Haberland V, Browne F, et al. Review of applications

of high-throughput sequencing in personalized medicine: Barriers and facilitators of future progress in research and clinical application. Briefings in Bioinformatics. 2019;**20**(5):1795-1811. DOI: 10.1093/bib/bby051

[15] Alterovitz G, Dean D, Goble C, et al. Enabling precision medicine via standard communication of HTS provenance, analysis, and results. PLoS Biology. 2018;**16**(12):e3000099. DOI: 10.1371/journal.pbio.3000099

[16] Jameson JL, Longo DL. Precision medicine—Personalized, problematic, and promising. The New England Journal of Medicine. 2015;**372**(23):2229-2234. DOI: 10.1056/NEJMsb1503104

[17] Phan N, Hong JJ, Tofig B, et al. A simple high-throughput approach identifies actionable drug sensitivities in patient-derived tumororganoids. Communications Biology. 2019;**2**:78. DOI: 10.1038/s42003-019-0305-x

[18] Wang ZG, Zhang L, Zhao WJ. Definition and application of precision medicine. Chinese Journal of Traumatology. 2016;**19**(5):249-250. DOI: 10.1016/j.cjtee.2016.04.005

[19] Hasanzad M, Sarhangi N, AghaeiMeybodi HR, Nikfar S, Khatami F, Larijani B. Precision medicine in non communicable diseases. International Journal of Molecular and Cellular Medicine. 2019;**8**(Suppl1):1-18. DOI: 10.22088/IJMCM.BUMS.8.2.1

[20] Wang C, Xu P, Zhang L, Huang J, Zhu K, Luo C. Current strategies and applications for precision drug design. Frontiers in Pharmacology. 2018;**9**:787. DOI: 10.3389/fphar.2018.00787

[21] Taylor JY, Barcelona de Mendoza V. Improving -omics-based research and precision health in minority populations: Recommendations for nurse scientists. Journal of Nursing Scholarship. 2018;**50**(1):11-19. DOI: 10.1111/jnu.12358

[22] Chen R, Mias GI, Li-Pook-Than J, et al. Personal omics profiling reveals dynamic molecular and medical phenotypes. Cell. 2012;**148**(6):1293-1307. DOI: 10.1016/j.cell.2012.02.009

[23] Rehm HL. Disease-targeted sequencing: A cornerstone in the clinic. Nature Reviews. Genetics. 2013;**14**(4):295-300. DOI: 10.1038/nrg3463

[24] Shyr D, Liu Q. Next generation sequencing in cancer research and clinical application. Biological Procedures Online. 2013;**15**(1):4. DOI: 10.1186/1480-9222-15-4

[25] Reuter JA, Spacek DV, Snyder MP. High-throughput sequencing technologies. Molecular Cell. 2015;**58**(4):586-597. DOI: 10.1016/j.molcel.2015.05.004

[26] Nussinov R, Jang H, Tsai CJ, Cheng F. Correction: Review: Precision medicine and driver mutations: Computational methods, functional assays and conformational principles for interpreting cancer drivers. PLoSComputational Biology. 2019;**15**(6):e1007114. DOI: 10.1371/journal.pcbi.1007114

[27] Zhu S, Rooney S, Michlewski G. RNA-targeted therapies and high-throughput screening methods. International Journal of Molecular Sciences. 2020;**21**(8):2996. DOI: 10.3390/ijms21082996

[28] Azarian T, Cook RL, Johnson JA, et al. Whole-genome sequencing for outbreak investigations of methicillin-resistant Staphylococcus aureus in the neonatal intensive care unit: Time for routine practice? Infection Control and Hospital Epidemiology. 2015;**36**(7):777-785. DOI: 10.1017/ice.2015.73

[29] Putignani L, Gasbarrini A, Dallapiccola B. Potential of multiomics technology in precision medicine. Current Opinion in Gastroenterology. 2019;**35**(6):491-498. DOI: 10.1097/MOG.0000000000000589

[30] Centers for disease control and prevention (CDC). Infectious Diseases: Precision Medicine for Public Health. 2022. https://blogs.cdc.gov/genomics/2015/09/24/infectious-diseases/ [Accessed: January 30, 2022]

[31] Lange C, Aarnoutse R, Chesov D, et al. Perspective for precision medicine for tuberculosis. Frontiers in Immunology. 2020;**11**:566608. DOI: 10.3389/fimmu.2020.566608

[32] Leguia M, Vila-Sanjurjo A, Chain PSG, Berry IM, Jarman RG, Pollett S. Precision medicine and precision public health in the era of pathogen next-generation sequencing. The Journal of Infectious Diseases. 2020;**221**(Suppl 3): S289-S291. DOI: 10.1093/infdis/jiz424

[33] Coffey DG, Cowan AJ, DeGraaff B, et al. High-throughput drug screening and multi-omic analysis to guide individualized treatment for multiple myeloma. JCO Precision Oncology. 2021;**5**:PO.20.00442. DOI: 10.1200/PO.20.00442

[34] Quartararo CE, Reznik E, deCarvalho AC, Mikkelsen T, Stockwell BR. High-throughput screening of patient-derived cultures reveals potential for precision medicine in glioblastoma. ACS Medical Chemistry Letters. 2015;**6**(8):948-952. DOI: 10.1021/acsmedchemlett.5b00128

[35] Tsoli M, Wadham C, Pinese M, et al. Integration of genomics, high throughput drug screening, and personalized xenograft models as a novel precision medicine paradigm for high risk pediatric cancer. Cancer Biology and Therapy. 2018;**19**(12): 1078-1087. DOI: 10.1080/15384047.2018.1491498

Section 2

High-Throughput Screening Based Drug Discovery for Infectious Diseases

Chapter 2

High-Throughput Screening for Drug Discovery toward Infectious Diseases: Options and Challenges

Ankur Gupta, Swatantra Kumar, Vimal K. Maurya, Bipin Puri and Shailendra K. Saxena

Abstract

The increase in the number of antibiotic-resistant microbial strains makes it evident to discover and develop newer efficacious anti-infective drugs. High-throughput screening (HTS) is a robust technology that plays a crucial role in identifying novel anti-infective lead compounds. This chapter briefly explains the role of virtual HTS (vHTS) and HTS technologies in lead identification using various categories of chemical libraries through structure-based drug design, ligand-based drug design, *in vitro* cell-based assay, and biochemical assay approaches involved in the process of drug design and discovery. The chapter also gives an insightful survey of the technologies such as fluorescence, luminescence, and atomic absorbance used for the detection of biological responses in the HTS bioassays. Applications of HTS, reverse pharmacology, current challenges, and future perspectives of HTS in the pharmaceutical and biotechnology industry are discussed in the context of anti-infective drug design, discovery, and development.

Keywords: HTS, vHTS, bioassay, anti-infective, drug discovery

1. Introduction

Antibiotic resistance among evolving microbes has been a matter of concern for pharmaceutical and biotechnology companies around the globe. These emerging pathogens with multiple drug resistance capabilities necessitate the discovery and development of both novel targets and anti-infective drugs. The key to success in anti-infective drug discovery depends on the identification of the target (a novel target for existing or novel strain of microbe) and a substantially active lead molecule against the designated target. Among the two key steps, the former requires genome sequence analysis (genomics) and protein expression analysis (proteomics) to identify target genes/proteins for a broad variety of microbial pathways and the latter requires chemical library screening against the defined target [1]. The chemical library may be generated through various routes such as combinatorial chemistry, bioassay-guided isolation of natural products, food and drug administration (FDA)-approved drugs for repurposing, virtually designed chemical library based on structure-based drug design (SBDD) or quantitative structure-activity relationship (QSAR), or other chemicals for fragment-based drug design (FBDD). However, with the latest advancement in technology, lead identification can be performed

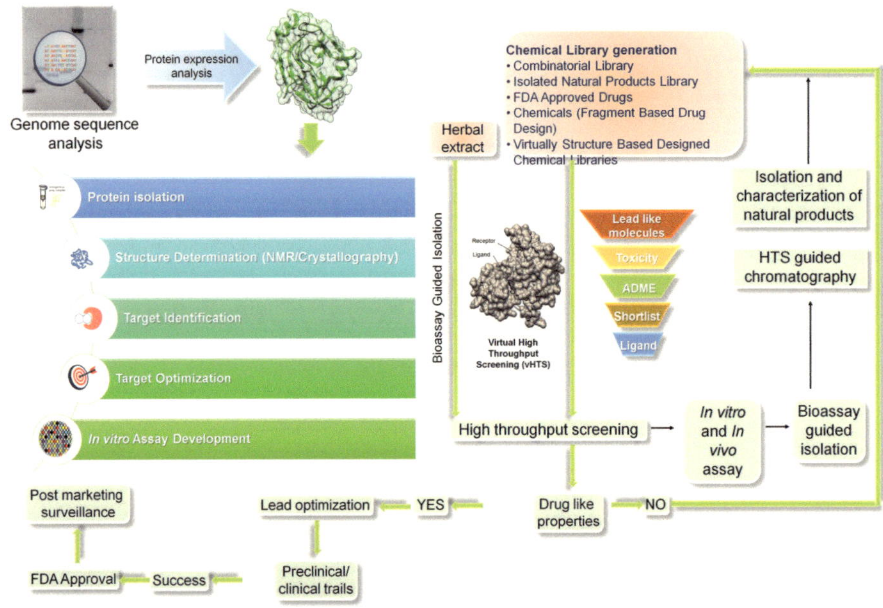

Figure 1.
Drug discovery process.

using high-throughput screening (HTS). HTS is a highly efficient automated method of screening chemical libraries to identify the so-called "hits," which are further modified to drug "leads" for lead optimization through medicinal chemistry approaches [2]. Generally, HTS involves biological or biochemical assay screening [3], whereas computer-based chemical library screening for "hits" identification is termed virtual high-throughput screening (vHTS). However, both the methods are used simultaneously or in parallel enabling the scientists to think computationally, act chemically, and observe biologically [4, 5]; therefore, in the present chapter, vHTS has been coupled with HTS for ease of understanding the correlation between all the stages of the drug discovery process (**Figure 1**).

2. HTS in drug discovery for infectious diseases

Infectious diseases arise in any person due to certain microbes which enter the body and multiply to give clinical symptoms of the disease. While some infections are contagious and spread from one person to another person, others may spread in the community through infectious vectors (insect/animal bites) or contaminated air, water, and food [6]. These microbes undergo mechanisms of resistance to antibiotics either under the direct influence of antibiotics or through adaptive processes unrelated to the chemical structures of antibiotics [7, 8]. The increase in the number of antibiotic-resistant microbial strains makes it evident to discover and develop newer efficacious drugs. However, developing a new drug is a tedious and complex process with uncertain outcomes; therefore, the process needs to be rational in approach. HTS offers a highly rationalized automation approach to explore large chemical space in a time-efficient manner. However, it requires complex and costly technological platforms which are generally available in pharmaceutical companies [4]. Nevertheless, it is not expensive because HTS screens a huge number of chemical compounds as compared to manual methods for target-to-lead discovery. An overall success rate of HTS to find leads is considered ~50%. However, vHTS is considered

DOI: http://dx.doi.org/10.5772/intechopen.102936

to have a higher success rate, but every method has its strengths and weaknesses, and therefore both the methods, HTS and vHTS, should be coupled for lead discovery. Few examples, among successful HTS drug discoveries in anti-infective agents, are (i) G-protein-coupled receptor (GPCR) inhibitor, Maraviroc (anti-HIV), (ii) reverse transcriptase (RT) inhibitor, etravirine (anti-HIV), [9] and (iii) hepatitis C virus (HCV) genotype 1a/b or 3 RNA replication inhibitor, Daclatasvir [10].

2.1 Need of HTS in drug discovery for infectious diseases

Bacterial enzymes play a significant role in developing antibiotic resistance through several key mechanisms and genetically derived mutations happening in: (i) drug-modifying enzymes (such as *transferases* and *hydrolases*), (ii) drug-metabolizing enzymes (such as *pyrazinamidase*, *catalase-peroxidase*, and *monooxygenase*), (iii) antibiotic's target enzymes (such as *RNA-dependent RNA polymerase* (RdRp) and *Topoisomerase II*), and (iv) antibiotic's cellular target-modifying enzymes (*rRNA-methyltransferases* and *phosphoethanolaminetransferase*). The structural changes in these enzymes not only lead to resistance among microbes but also open the 'omics gates to identify newer targets that originated after modifications in enzymes [8–10]. The rapid spread of resistance among microbes makes it imperative to rapidly identify new classes of antibiotics. Traditionally, growth inhibition assays are used for antimicrobial drug discovery which is a slow process [11, 12]. However, to match the pace of microbial resistance to antibiotics, a robotic automation screening process with efficient, accurate, and robust scientific methodology is required. HTS offers an economic advantage of screening huge chemical spaces accurately within defined timelines. Therefore, time, cost, and quality are termed as the "magic triangle of HTS" [13]. The credit of rapid HTS goes to: (i) high-density arrays, micro-reaction wells, and (ii) biological response detection methods.

High-density array micro-reaction well plates ranging from 96-well plates to miniaturized 3456-well plates are available with typical working volumes ranging from 1 to 10 μl of total volume. However, efforts are being made for further miniaturization of plates [13] to develop mega-dense arrays (>10,000 wells/plate) [14]. Although there are few difficulties associated with ultra-high-density plates, nevertheless, it is possible to perform 100,000 assays per day using ultra-high-throughput screening (uHTS) [15].

Biological response detection techniques such as fluorescence, luminescence, and atomic absorption spectroscopy have been established, which makes the process robust in the identification of active compounds. These direct and indirect detection methods have been developed based on: (i) direct measurement of absorbance and (ii) indirect measurement through enzymatic or chemical reactions coupled with pH indicators and chelators. These methods establish a quantitative relationship between biological response and target metabolite concentration [16]. Apart from the pharmacological aspect, HTS is equally beneficial in the evaluation of toxicological aspects of the chemical entities such as (i) genotoxicity, (ii) carcinogenicity, and (iii) immunotoxicity [15].

Plants have an abundance of potentially diverse chemical entities in the form of complex mixtures which are required to be evaluated in HTS for the discovery of new drugs against microbes. However, pure chemical entities from these complex mixtures need to be isolated and structurally characterized before proceeding for target-specific evaluation. Bioassay (*in vitro*)-guided HTS of these plant extracts aids in the identification and isolation of bioactive compounds (**Figure 1**) [17].

Similarly, vHTS is a bioethical approach consisting of a wide variety of *in silico* simulation approaches to explore chemical libraries and identify which chemical entity has the potential to display *in vitro* and/or *in vivo* drug-like properties in HTS. However, there are chances of false-negative and false-positive results [4].

3. Methods involved in HTS for drug discovery toward infectious diseases

3.1 Classification of HTS

HTS methods for anti-infective drug discovery may be biological (cell-based or whole organism), biochemical (enzymes/receptors), and virtual (computer-based). Hence, the HTS methods may be classified as summarized in **Figure 2**. The HTS assay approach for the identification of "lead" molecule may vary depending on the target; however, the assay protocol must be (i) sensitive to low potency molecules, (ii) reproducible in biological response, (iii) accurate in terms of positive and negative control, and (iv) economically feasible. Therefore, these parameters should be optimized before proceeding with the assay of compounds in large numbers [18].

3.1.1 Virtual high-throughput screening (computer simulation-guided selection)

vHTS is an efficient approach to identify hits and lead compounds for an identified microbial target which are further optimized using medicinal chemistry approaches. The applications of vHTS can be further explored to virtually evaluate ADMET (absorption, distribution, metabolism, excretion, and toxicity) properties of the identified lead chemical entities based on "Lipinski's rule." The shortlisted potential hit/lead molecules may then be evaluated *in vitro,* thus giving a meaningful rationale between computer simulations and practical experimentation. Where vHTS is a generalized term for different screening filters, it is categorized under two broad classes of virtual screening methods. These methods are (i) structure-based drug design (SBDD) and ligand-based drug design (LBDD) [19].

3.1.1.1 Structure-based drug design

Advances in HT 'omics technologies and instrumental methods of analysis such as X-ray crystallography and nuclear magnetic resonance (NMR) have solved a large number of three-dimensional (3D) structures of target proteins involved in communicable and noncommunicable diseases. These structures with specific identification numbers and resolution are available for scientific research and education purposes in protein data bank (PDB) [20]. Therefore, understanding the biologically functional interacting pocket (druggable target site) within 3D structures of the target proteins is essential to proceed with SBDD. However, if this structural information is not completely reliable or any sequence of the structural information is missing, then homology modeling is performed to generate a homologous model of the target protein [21]. SBDD is further classified under two headings; (i) docking and scoring and (ii) *de novo* drug design.

Docking and scoring is an excellent approach to predict the binding affinity and pharmacodynamic status of small chemical entities (ligands) in the active site of the target macromolecule. Scoring is an energy function which estimates the free binding energy of protein-ligand interactions such as electrostatic and van der Waals forces. Docking may be performed using two theoretical strategies namely: (i) lock and key theory, and (ii) induced-fit theory. Earlier docking programs were run using the lock and key assumptions where both the target protein and the ligand were treated as rigid structures with docking affinity dependent on the shape of the

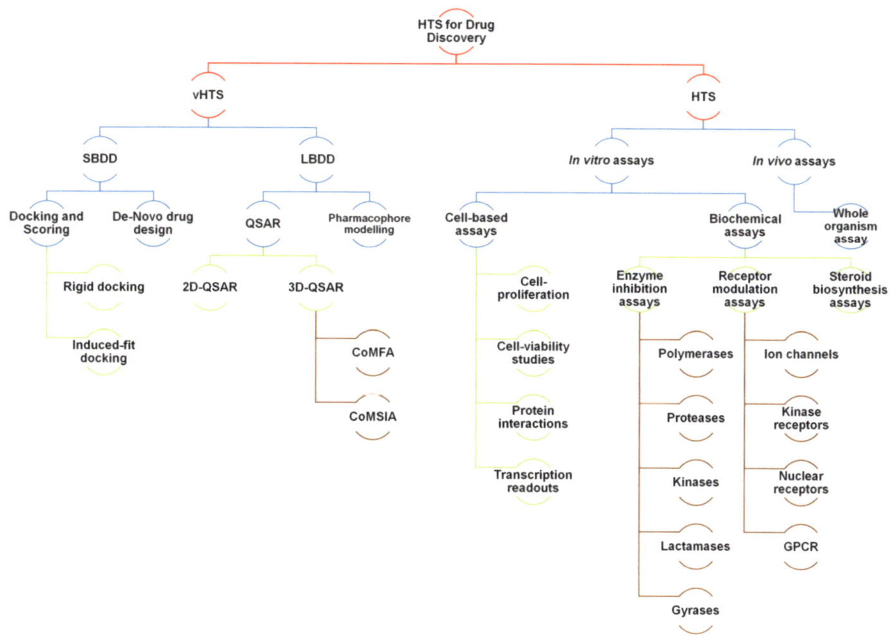

Figure 2.
Classification of HTS for anti-infective drug discovery.

interacting structures. Hence, it is termed as a rigid docking program. However, the target proteins and ligands are never in their rigid conformational state; instead, they are flexible (induced-fit docking) and undertake complementary conformational changes. Therefore, optimizing the binding pocket enables it to accommodate ligands of various shapes and sizes. This approach reduces the dropping out chances of potential false negatives [22, 23].

De novo design is a method of drug design that involves six different strategies: (i) identifying site point within the target site and connecting them using chemical fragments, (ii) determination of desirable fragment location, (iii) positioning fragment within the target site and linking them with linkers or scaffolds, (iv) construction of ligand sequentially within the site using fragments, (v) whole molecule conformation and interaction studies similar to docking, and (vi) random connection methods [24].

3.1.1.2 Ligand-based drug design

LBDD approach is applicable when nothing is known about the 3D structure of the target site and completely relies on the knowledge of previously established lead/drug molecules with known pharmacological/toxicological profiles and 2D/3D physicochemical descriptors. Therefore, LBDD is classified into two broad categories: (i) quantitative structure–activity relationship (QSAR) [25] and (ii) pharmacophore modeling [26]. However, scaffold hopping [27] and pseudo-receptor modeling [28] are also the strategies used in LBDD.

QSAR is a method for developing mathematical models to significantly correlate the pharmacological profile with the chemical structures within the data set using regression analysis. However, with technological advancement, the QSAR method has undergone dimensional transformations (2D and 3D). The process involves a collection of chemical data sets (in-house or external) to develop mathematical QSAR models. These models are then used to identify active compounds which are sequentially evaluated and synthesized on various platforms, including docking, *in vitro*, and *in vivo* studies [25].

Scaffold hopping is also known as "lead hopping" as it starts with known active compounds which are modified using 1–4° chemical replacement in the known lead structure to generate a novel chemotype which is further evaluated using various platforms, including docking, *in vitro*, and *in vivo* studies [27]. In contrast, pseudo-receptor design is a method closely related to homology modeling of SBDD where presumed bioactive conformations of overlaid molecules are used to generate the target's pseudo-binding site map for further SBDD. Hence, this method is a bridge between LBDD and SBDD [28].

Pharmacophore fingerprinting is a method to identify a common "pharmacophore feature" among a set of active drug or lead molecules that may be used in SBDD and/or LBDD. The pharmacophore feature is an essential chemical portion of lead/drug molecules which is required for biological functions and may include hydrogen bond donors/acceptors, aromatic rings, hydrophilic/hydrophobic attachments, or any possible combinations. These features are enumerated in terms of three-point and four-point sets of varied pharmacophores to measure the distance in terms of bonds. Pharmacophore fingerprints thus generated are utilized for developing novel lead molecules in combination with SBDD (**Figure 3**) [26].

3.1.2 High-throughput screening (bioassay-guided selection)

3.1.2.1 Cell-based assays

Various unexplored targets and pathways lie within the components of cellular complexity which offers an excellent platform to identify antimicrobial lead molecules through the cell (or organism)-based HTS. Thus, multiple targets can be screened using cell-based assays in all the stages of drug discovery. In simple words, these assays are used when the desired cellular target is either unknown or the

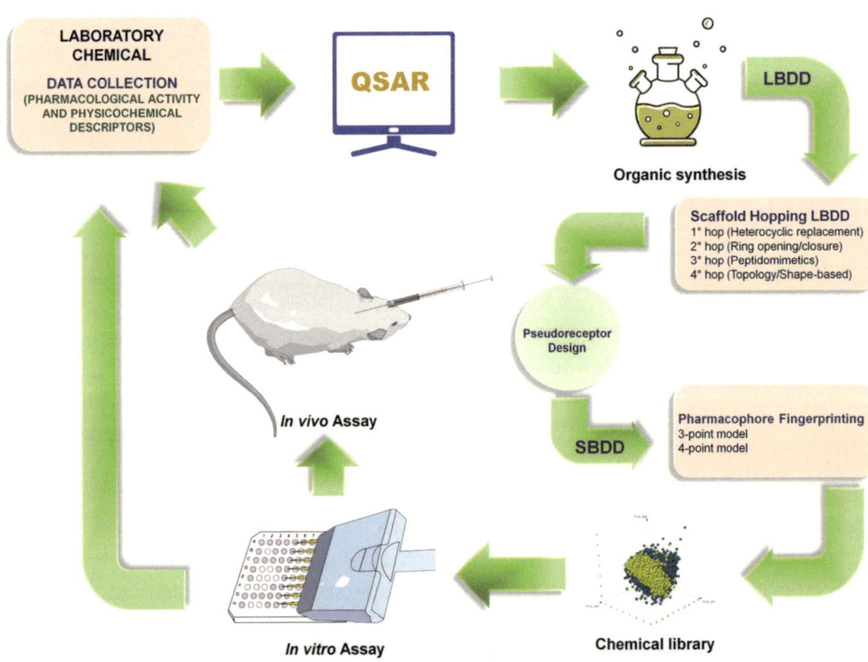

Figure 3.
Ligand and structure-based drug designing process.

phenotype cannot be separated from the cellular context. Nevertheless, these assays provide additional information which cannot be obtained from biochemical assays or vHTS, such as membrane permeability, pharmacodynamic (agonist, partial agonist, inverse agonist, and antagonist) status, cell proliferation (or viability), cytotoxicity, heterogeneity, protein expression, transcriptional readouts, and phenotypic biomarker readouts. Thus, cell-based assays may be classified depending on the methodologies used such as: (i) cell viability assays using (a.) dyes like Alamar blue, tetrazolium compounds (MTT assay, XTT assay, and MTS assay) which get converted to generate fluorescence or color indicating cell death or viability; (b.) luciferin-luciferase assay where ATP content is measured using luciferin-luciferase to generate bioluminescence; (c.) intercalation with membrane-permeant DNA dyes; (ii) reporter gene assay; (iii) secondary messenger assay; (iv) protein-fragment complementation assay; (v) protein–protein interaction assay; (vi) label-free methods; and (vii) phenotype biomarker assays. For anti-infective drug discovery, cell viability assays with different cell lines are utilized to screen and identify molecules that can kill or inhibit the growth of pathogens. These assays are further utilized to evaluate the safety issues of the organs such as the liver because the liver is the primary center for drug metabolism [29].

3.1.2.2 Biochemical assays

Biochemical assays involve screening of chemical libraries for *in vitro* inhibition of purified target protein (enzyme, receptor, and ion channels) in competition format where the known substrate bound to protein is replaced by the ligand or compound under study. The biological response is detected using optical methods such as fluorescence, luminescence, or absorbance [29].

3.2 Biological response detection methods in HTS

The detection of biological response in the cell-based and/or biochemical assay may be performed using different analytical technologies such as, fluorescence-based assays [FRET, HTRF, dissociation-enhanced lanthanide fluorescent immunoassay (DELFIA), time-resolved FRET (TR-FRET), fluorescence polarization (FP), fluorescent lifetime (FLT)], luminescence-based assays [bioluminescence resonance energy transfer (BRET), amplified luminescent proximity homogeneous assay (ALPHA), electrochemiluminescence assay (ECL)], atomic absorption spectroscopy (AAS), high-throughput electrophysiology (HT electrophysiology), protein complementation assay (PCA), Scintillation proximity assay (SPA), and enzyme fragment complementation (EFC) [18], which are further modified with different variations. However, the detailed discussion on the usage of these variations in the design of HTS assays is beyond the scope of this chapter.

4. Applications and outcomes of HTS in anti-infective drug discovery

HTS is being applied in a myriad of ways starting from the biology of infectious diseases to finding the lead molecules for anti-infective drug discovery. Few applications of HTS in infectious biology are the identification of pathogenic molecular mechanisms, evolutionary analysis of pathogens, and determination of the determinants required for survival and pathogenesis of the mutant strains of the microbial population [30]. Although, HTS is an early-stage drug development program, however, the anti-infective drug discovery efforts with HTS from the year 2000 to date have led to the approval of 38 new antibacterial drugs and 67 drug candidates are in the clinical development stage for both Gram-negative and Gram-positive bacteria including *Mycobacterium tuberculosis*. Nevertheless, 19 different compounds with novel pharmacophore are in different stages of clinical development (6 compounds in Phase I, 9 compounds in Phase II, 4 compounds in Phase III) [31].

5. Reverse pharmacology in drug discovery for infectious diseases

HTS bioassay-guided identification and isolation of bioactive compounds from natural biodiversity is termed as "Reverse Pharmacognosy." Similarly, isolating a chemical entity and developing a pharmaceutical product from the clinically proven herbal remedy is termed "Reverse Pharmacology." Quinine and Artemisinin are the two well-known antimalarial lead molecules identified and isolated through this approach [32] which were optimized using HTS and chemistry approaches to various antimalarial drugs with a better pharmacokinetic and pharmacodynamic profile.

6. Challenges in drug discovery for infectious diseases

The major challenge in drug discovery for infectious diseases is the mutation in superbugs which make them evolve rapidly. Despite the availability of structural information of 62,206 bacterially derived proteins in PDB, mutational changes in these structures necessitate continuous research in 'omics studies. Moreover, the virus-derived proteins are only 9603 in number [20] leading to a reduced success rate of structure-based design of antiviral drugs. Nevertheless, many QSAR projects fail at the model building stage due to a lack of interdisciplinary application during the execution of the project. Similarly, a considerable challenge at the stage of *in vitro/in vivo* screening is the penetration of molecules into the bacterial cell, especially in Gram-negative species. However, these challenges may be countered with a diversified chemical space which is again a challenge for combinatorial chemistry-based chemical libraries. Therefore, biodiversity needs to be explored for identifying novel pharmacophores and associated anti-infective drugs.

7. Future perspectives

Highly diversified chemical space is a must for identifying novel pharmacophores which can be obtained through engineering biodiversity. Phytochemical hybridization [33] and phytochemical engineering [34] offer a great advantage to generate diverse semisynthetic chemical libraries which may be fruitful in identifying novel anti-infective pharmacophores. Further, nanotechnology is an emerging technology through which nanoprobes may be utilized to analyze microbes. Hence, HTS incorporated with nanotechnology may improve the efficiency of HTS [16]. Similarly, microfluidic technology may enable the use of a single platform to combine genome sequencing, mining, and uHTS. Thus, this technology may open up unique opportunities for anti-infective drug discovery at the level of single cell [35]. Further, given the urgency of the coronavirus (CoV) outbreak, HTS methodology using two types of mild CoV, HCoV-OC43 and MHV, was developed as a valuable tool for the rapid identification of promising drugs against CoV without the drawbacks of level three biological confinements. The luciferase reporter gene is introduced into HCoV-OC43 and MHV to indicate viral activity, and hence the antiviral efficiency of screened drugs can be quantified by luciferase activity. Compounds with antiviral activity against both HCoV-OC43 and MHV are further evaluated in SARS-CoV-2 after structural optimizations. This system allows large-scale compounds to be screened to search for broad spectrum drugs against CoV in a high-throughput manner, providing potential alternatives for clinical management of SARS-CoV-2 [36].

8. Conclusions

The goal of this chapter was to elucidate various options and platforms of the drug discovery process in correlation with anti-infective drugs. Where most of the discovery aspects starting from microbial resistance to target-to-lead identification through HTS strategies such as structure-based, ligand-based drug design, *in vitro* cell-based/biochemical assays, and biological response detection techniques are covered, the detailed explanation on each subtopic may be referred using the reference section. However, the challenges in anti-infective drug discovery remain a matter of concern for future research and development using different techniques to generate chemical space such as phytochemical hybridization and incorporation of nanotechnology in HTS for ultra-efficient screening and detection of biological response.

Acknowledgements

The authors are grateful to: the Director-General, Department of Health & Family Welfare, Government of Sikkim, India; the Principal, Government Pharmacy College, Sikkim, India; and the Vice-Chancellor, King George's Medical University (KGMU), Lucknow, India, for the support and encouragement for this work.

Conflict of interest

The authors declare no conflict of interest.

Author details

Ankur Gupta[1†], Swatantra Kumar[2], Vimal K. Maurya[2], Bipin Puri[2] and Shailendra K. Saxena[2*†]

1 Government Pharmacy College, Sajong, Rumtek, Sikkim, India

2 Centre for Advanced Research (CFAR), Faculty of Medicine, King George's Medical University (KGMU), Lucknow, India

*Address all correspondence to: shailen@kgmcindia.edu

† These authors contributed equally to this work as first author.

References

[1] Doostparast Torshizi A, Wang K. Next-generation sequencing in drug development: Target identification and genetically stratified clinical trials. Drug Discovery Today. 2018;**23**(10):1776-1783. DOI: 10.1016/j.drudis.2018.05.015

[2] Payne DJ, Gwynn MN, Holmes DJ, Pompliano DL. Drugs for bad bugs: Confronting the challenges of antibacterial discovery. Nature Reviews. Drug Discovery. 2007;**6**(1):29-40. DOI: 10.1038/nrd2201

[3] Aldewachi H, Al-Zidan RN, Conner MT, Salman MM. High-throughput screening platforms in the discovery of novel drugs for neurodegenerative diseases. Bioengineering (Basel). 2021;**8**(2):30. DOI: 10.3390/bioengineering8020030

[4] Bellera CL, Sbaraglini ML, Talevi A. Modern approaches for the discovery of anti-infectious drugs for the treatment of neglected diseases. Current Topics in Medicinal Chemistry. 2018;**18**(5):369-381. DOI: 10.2174/156802661866618 0509151146

[5] Johnson EO, Hung DT. A point of inflection and reflection on systems chemical biology. ACS Chemical Biology. 2019;**14**(12):2497-2511. DOI: 10.1021/acschembio.9b00714

[6] National Center for Emerging and Zoonotic Infectious Diseases. Available from: https://www.cdc.gov/ncezid/pdf/ncezid_brochure_2012.pdf [Accessed: June 21, 2021].

[7] Holmes AH, Moore LS, Sundsfjord A, et al. Understanding the mechanisms and drivers of antimicrobial resistance. Lancet. 2016;**387**(10014):176-187. DOI: 10.1016/S0140-6736(15)00473-0

[8] Egorov AM, Ulyashova MM, Rubtsova MY. Bacterial enzymes and antibiotic resistance. ActaNaturae. 2018;**10**(4):33-48

[9] Macarron R, Banks MN, Bojanic D, et al. Impact of high-throughput screening in biomedical research. Nature Reviews. Drug Discovery. 2011;**10**(3): 188-195. DOI: 10.1038/nrd3368

[10] Available from: https://www.drugs.com/history/daklinza.html [Accessed: June 21 2021]

[11] Projan SJ, Shlaes DM. Antibacterial drug discovery: is it all downhill from here? Clinical Microbiology and Infection. 2004;**4**(Suppl. 10):18-22. DOI: 10.1111/j.1465-0691.2004.1006.x

[12] Silver LL. A retrospective on the failures and successes of antibacterial drug discovery. IDrugs. 2005;**8**(8): 651-655

[13] Mayr LM, Fuerst P. The future of high-throughput screening. Journal of Biomolecular Screening. 2008;**13**(6): 443-448. DOI: 10.1177/108705710 8319644

[14] Wingren C, Borrebaeck CA. Progress in miniaturization of protein arrays-a step closer to high-density nanoarrays. Drug Discovery Today. 2007;**12**(19-20):813-819. DOI: 10.1016/j.drudis.2007.08.003

[15] Szymański P, Markowicz M, Mikiciuk-Olasik E. Adaptation of high-throughput screening in drug discovery-toxicological screening tests. International Journal of Molecular Sciences. 2012;**13**(1):427-452. DOI: 10.3390/ijms13010427

[16] Zeng W, Guo L, Xu S, Chen J, Zhou J. High-throughput screening technology in industrial biotechnology. Trends in Biotechnology. 2020;**38**(8): 888-906. DOI: 10.1016/j.tibtech.2020.01.001

[17] Zhang HJ, Li WF, Fong HH, Soejarto DD. Discovery of bioactive compounds by the uic-icbg drug discovery program in the 18 years since 1998. Molecules. 2016;**21**(11):1448. DOI: 10.3390/molecules21111448

[18] Inglese J, Johnson RL, Simeonov A, et al. High-throughput screening assays for the identification of chemical probes. Nature Chemical Biology. 2007;**3**(8):466-479. DOI: 10.1038/nchembio.2007.17

[19] Aparoy P, Reddy KK, Reddanna P. Structure and ligand-based drug design strategies in the development of novel 5- LOX inhibitors. Current Medicinal Chemistry. 2012;**19**(22):3763-3778. DOI: 10.2174/092986712801661112

[20] Available from: Protein data bank. https://www.rcsb.org/ [Accessed: June 21, 2021].

[21] Muhammed MT, Aki-Yalcin E. Homology modeling in drug discovery: Overview, current applications, and future perspectives. Chemical Biology & Drug Design. 2019;**93**(1):12-20. DOI: 10.1111/cbdd.13388

[22] Gazgalis D, Zaka M, Abbasi BH, Logothetis DE, Mezei M, Cui M. Protein binding pocket optimization for virtual high-throughput screening (vHTS) drug discovery. ACS Omega. 2020;**5**(24):14297-14307. DOI: 10.1021/acsomega.0c00522

[23] Badrinarayan P, Sastry GN. Virtual high throughput screening in new lead identification. Combinatorial Chemistry & High Throughput Screening. 2011;**14**(10):840-860. DOI: 10.2174/138620711797537102

[24] Murcko MA. In: Lipkowitz KB, Boyd DB, editors. Reviews in Computational Chemistry. Vol. 11. Hoboken, NJ, USA: John Wiley & Sons, Inc.; 2007. pp. 1-67

[25] Neves BJ, Braga RC, Melo-Filho CC, Moreira-Filho JT, Muratov EN, Andrade CH. QSAR-based virtual screening: Advances and applications in drug discovery. Frontiers in Pharmacology. 2018;**9**:1275. DOI: 10.3389/fphar.2018.01275

[26] Qing X, Lee XY, De Raeymaecker J, et al. Pharmacophoremodeling: advances, limitations, and current utility in drug discovery. Journal of Receptor, Ligand and Channel Research. 2014;7:81-92. DOI: 10.2147/JRLCR.S46843

[27] Sun H, Tawa G, Wallqvist A. Classification of scaffold-hopping approaches. Drug Discovery Today. 2012;**17**(7-8):310-324. DOI: 10.1016/j.drudis.2011.10.024

[28] Fayne D. Ligand-based molecular design using pseudoreceptors. In: Schneider G, editor. Chapter 9 De Novo Molecular Design. Germany: Wiley; 2013. pp. 227-244. DOI: 10.1002/9783527677016.ch9

[29] Blay V, Tolani B, Ho SP, Arkin MR. High-throughput screening: Today's biochemical and cell-based approaches. Drug Discovery Today. 2020;**S1359-6446**(20):30305-30306. DOI: 10.1016/j.drudis.2020.07.024

[30] McAdam PR, Richardson EJ, Fitzgerald JR. High-throughput sequencing for the study of bacterial pathogen biology. Current Opinion in Microbiology. 2014;**19**(100):106-113. DOI: 10.1016/j.mib.2014.06.002

[31] Butler MS, Paterson DL. Antibiotics in the clinical pipeline in October 2019. The Journal of Antibiotics (Tokyo). 2020;**73**(6):329-364. DOI: 10.1038/s41429-020-0291-8

[32] Willcox ML, Graz B, Falquet J, Diakite C, Giani S, Diallo D. A reverse pharmacology approach for developing an anti-malarial phytomedicine. Malaria Journal. 2011;**10**(Suppl. 1):S8. DOI: 10.1186/1475-2875-10-S1-S8

[33] Swain SS, Paidesetty SK, Padhy RN. Phytochemical conjugation as a potential semisynthetic approach toward reactive and reuse of obsolete sulfonamides against pathogenic bacteria. Drug Development Research. 2021;**82**(2):149-166. DOI: 10.1002/ddr.21746

[34] Muhammad A, Feng X, Rasool A, Sun W, Li C. Production of plant natural products through engineered Yarrowialipolytica. Biotechnology Advances. 2020;**43**:107555. DOI: 10.1016/j.biotechadv.2020.107555

[35] Terekhov SS, Osterman IA, Smirnov IV. High-throughput screening of biodiversity for antibiotic discovery. ActaNaturae. 2018;**10**(3):23-29

[36] Liu J, Li K, Cheng L, Shao J, Yang S, Zhang W, et al. A high-throughput drug screening strategy against coronaviruses. International Journal of Infectious Diseases. 2021;**103**:300-304. DOI: 10.1016/j.ijid.2020.12.033

Section 3

High-Throughput Screening for Novel Drug Designing/ Development

Chapter 3

Unbiased Identification of Extracellular Protein–Protein Interactions for Drug Target and Biologic Drug Discovery

Shengya Cao and Nadia Martinez-Martin

Abstract

Technological improvements in unbiased screening have accelerated drug target discovery. In particular, membrane-embedded and secreted proteins have gained attention because of their ability to orchestrate intercellular communication. Dysregulation of their extracellular protein–protein interactions (ePPIs) underlies the initiation and progression of many human diseases. Practically, ePPIs are also accessible for modulation by therapeutics since they operate outside of the plasma membrane. Therefore, it is unsurprising that while these proteins make up about 30% of human genes, they encompass the majority of drug targets approved by the FDA. Even so, most secreted and membrane proteins remain uncharacterized in terms of binding partners and cellular functions. To address this, a number of approaches have been developed to overcome challenges associated with membrane protein biology and ePPI discovery. This chapter will cover recent advances that use high-throughput methods to move towards the generation of a comprehensive network of ePPIs in humans for future targeted drug discovery.

Keywords: drug discovery, high-throughput screening, extracellular protein–protein interactions, unbiased target discovery, receptors, membrane proteins, secreted proteins

1. Introduction: targeting ePPIs to address disease burden

The World Health Organization estimates that over 70% of deaths in 2016 worldwide were due to non-communicable diseases like cardiovascular disease (CVD) and cancer. This number is expected to grow to over 80% by 2060 [1]. Even if these diseases arise from environmental damage, the disease states usually depend on altered cellular communication, driven at the molecular level by altered ePPIs. For example, interactions between immune cells and arterial walls through adhesion proteins can initiate positive feedback loops which drive atherosclerotic plaque formation in CVD [2]. Similarly, while genetic mutations are the root cause of cancer, aberrant cell–cell interactions allow cancer cells to evade the immune system [3], migrate [4], siphon nutrients [5] and ignore signals to stop growing [6]. EPPIs also contribute to communicable diseases, which, highlighted by the (ongoing as of this writing) COVID-19 pandemic, can rapidly increase human deaths with the introduction of a novel pathogen. As with many pathogens, the virus underlying the pandemic, SARS-CoV-2, exploits host cell-surface receptors to enter cells to replicate and spread [7, 8].

Because ePPIs are often central to the initiation and progression of diseases, they offer opportunities for molecular intervention using drugs. Greater understanding of the ePPIs underlying diseases allows them to be effectively targeted and manipulated to reverse disease phenotypes. For example, for CVD, several efforts to target different cytokines are showing promise in stemming the progression of atherosclerosis [9]. The development of cancer immunotherapies in the last decade has revolutionized cancer treatment. These treatments block ePPIs between immune checkpoint proteins such as CTLA-4 or PD-L1 and their binding partners to reinvigorate the body's defenses [10]. Even with SARS-CoV-2, an antibody cocktail (REGN-COV2) that blocks the ePPI between the virus spike protein and receptors on the cell, has been shown to stop viral entry and has gained emergency authorization for use in COVID-19 patients [11]. These examples highlight that identifying and targeting ePPIs can have strong therapeutic benefits in a variety of known and emerging diseases that make up a significant portion of human disease burden worldwide (**Figure 1**).

Despite the importance of ePPIs for both understanding and treating disease, our understanding of this field remains limited, especially compared to other classes of protein–protein interactions (PPIs). A main reason for this disparity is that common techniques for general PPI discovery are not well suited for ePPIs. Interactions between individual secreted or membrane proteins are typically weak, making them difficult to capture. Membrane proteins are biochemically recalcitrant and tend to misfold or aggregate outside of a native membrane context making them incompatible with many readouts designed for soluble proteins. Extracellular proteins also pick up many complex and heterogeneous post-translational modifications on their journey out of the cell, including specific disulfide bonds designed for the non-reducing extracellular environment. Since these can play roles in ePPIs but are not well characterized, they can be missed by common non-native expression

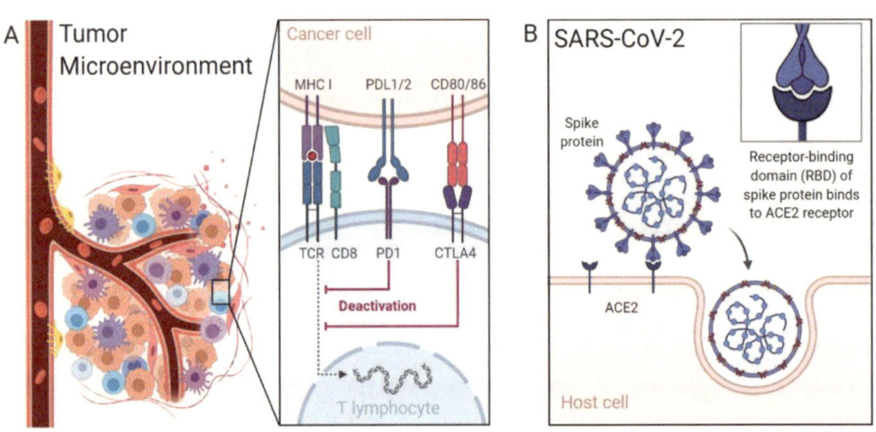

Figure 1.
Examples of therapeutically relevant ePPIs. (A) The tumor microenvironment consists of a complex mix of cell types that communicate through ePPIs. One example is the expression of immune checkpoint proteins such as PD-L1 on cancer cells, which inhibits cytotoxic T-cell function, allowing the cancer cells to evade the immune system. Drugs targeting these ePPIs are the foundation for the cancer immunotherapies, which have provided significant benefits for cancer patients. Many other ePPIs in this space are under active investigation. (B) SAR-CoV-2 uses its spike protein to co-op the ACE2 receptor for viral entry into host cells and initiate viral replication and infection. Strategies for blocking this interaction are being explored to address the COVID-19 pandemic.

systems [12, 13]. Altogether, these biochemical features make most available technologies suboptimal and as a result, ePPIs are remarkably underrepresented in current databases.

Because of the difficulties with ePPI discovery, many new approaches have been developed to specifically identify human ePPIs that play roles in homeostasis and disease. While past low-throughput methods and focused studies have provided fundamental insights into specific receptors and pathways, the rapid explosion in sequencing, mass spectrometry (MS), targeted mutagenesis and high-throughput screening techniques has made the exhaustive identification of ePPIs a realistic goal. Here, we will address how new techniques deal with unique challenges associated with ePPIs and highlight the progress towards to the elucidation of a comprehensive network map of all human ePPIs.

2. Methods for detecting ePPIs

From biophysical approaches to *in vivo* studies, a number of methods have been developed or are being improved that have the potential to enable unbiased ePPIs discovery. The majority of methods can be categorized into a few broad technological concepts: biochemical fractionation, affinity purification, protein-fragment complementation, proximity labeling, direct protein interaction detection and computational modeling. As is the case for other disciplines, deciphering the complexities of extracellular interactions requires a multipronged approach. Since the different approaches provide different types of information, these methodologies are complementary. Especially as these categories have matured, many new techniques bridge the different concepts to balance the various benefits and shortcomings and push for increased throughput. The specific method-of-choice will depend on the expertise, equipment and overall resources available in each laboratory (**Table 1**).

Approach	**Direct Interaction**	**Weak Interaction Detection**	**Correct Modification**	**Automation Preferred**	**False +**	**False –**
Biochemical Fractionation	Variable	+	+++	No	++	+++
Affinity Purification	+	+	+++	Variable	++	+++
Protein-fragment comple-mentation	++	++	++	Yes	++	++
Proximity labeling	+	+++	++	No	+++	+
Direct interaction screens	+++	++ – +++	+ – +++	Yes	+	+++

Table 1.
Comparison of approaches for unbiased detecting ePPIs.

2.1 Biochemical fractionation

2.1.1 Concept description

Biochemical fractionation is the splitting of a complex lysate, typically cell or tissue extract, into simpler mixtures to identify the simplest solution that retains a certain biochemical property. The measurable property could be complex cellular activities, such as the stimulation of cell migration, or simple ones such as binding to a target protein (**Figure 2**).

2.1.2 Concept pros

Biochemical fractionation does not require any knowledge of the components and can be an unbiased technique. It is a versatile concept since any biochemical property can be studied, from *in vivo* tissue level responses to molecular PPIs. Some degree of fractionation is easily combined with other techniques to reduce the starting complexity and to improve data interpretability.

2.1.3 Concept cons

The results from biochemical fractionations are dependent on the particular purification steps used and can be highly variable. Due to the multiple purification steps, this approach can also be labor and time intensive. The different purification steps can inactivate proteins by inducing misfolding or removing key co-factors. This is especially true for ePPIs that involve membrane proteins, which can lose activity if extracted from membranes [12, 13].

2.1.4 Specific applications

Biochemical fractionations played a role historically in identifying some of the first extracellular signaling proteins like cytokines using activities such as macrophage migration or bacteria killing [14]. In the 21st century, this approach has identified stable soluble PPIs proteome-wide by fractionating cell lysates down to the level of co-eluting protein complexes and identifying them using MS [15]. While the specific purification steps used for soluble proteins are unlikely to be applicable to ePPIs, alternative centrifugation-based fractionation successfully recovered biochemically active membranes from crude fruit fly extracts [16]. Direct application of affinity purification from crude extracts without enriching for synaptic membranes did not recover known ePPIs [16]. However, using biochemical fractionation to enrich for synaptic components was necessary for the identification of key proteins in synapse formation using an affinity purification approach (described in the next section) [17].

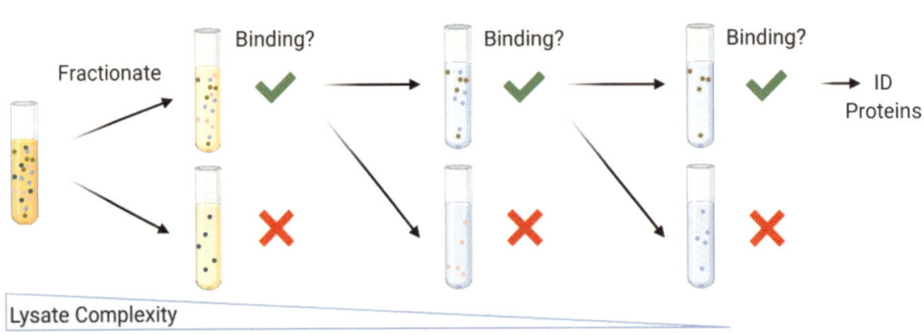

Figure 2.
Biochemical fractionation can be used to reduce the complexity of a mixture while maintaining the desired activity. While traditionally performed in series, fractionation can also be done in parallel with modern purification techniques.

DOI: http://dx.doi.org/10.5772/intechopen.97310

2.2 Affinity purification

2.2.1 Concept description

Affinity purification involves isolating a target-of-interest in non-denaturing conditions to enable co-isolation of any binding partners that are stably attached. The most common implementation is immunoprecipitation, where an antibody, generally attached to a solid substrate like a bead, plate or column, is used to specifically recognize the target-of-interest. Any factors that are not stably bound to the protein of interest are washed away by flushing the solid substrate with buffer. Proteins that survive the washes are identified (**Figure 3**).

2.2.2 Concept pros

Affinity purification allows for the direct isolation of a target-of-interest from complex mixtures. It is versatile and can be combined with many other approaches.

2.2.3 Concept cons

To isolate the target-of-interest, there needs to be a reagent, like an antibody, that will specifically and tightly bind the target. Since such reagents are not always readily available, the target may need to be tagged and introduced exogenously, which can affect target behavior. Affinity purification for unbiased identification of binding partners requires either large tagged libraries or access to MS. Importantly, to be identified, binding partners need to survive cell lysis and washes. This has limited the applicability of this otherwise widely-utilized approach in the study of ePPIs. Cell lysis and target extractions typically require membrane solubilization, which can disrupt membrane protein-dependent interactions. In addition, affinity purification workflows often miss detection of low affinity interactions, which are typical of ePPIs.

2.2.4 Specific applications

The most widely used version of this concept is affinity purification followed by binding partner identification using mass spectrometry (AP/MS) (**Table 2**). MS allows for the unbiased identification of interactors in their endogenous form in virtually any cell type or tissue. Traditionally, AP/MS studies were mostly restricted to one or a few targets-of-interest. However, recent technological advances, dominated

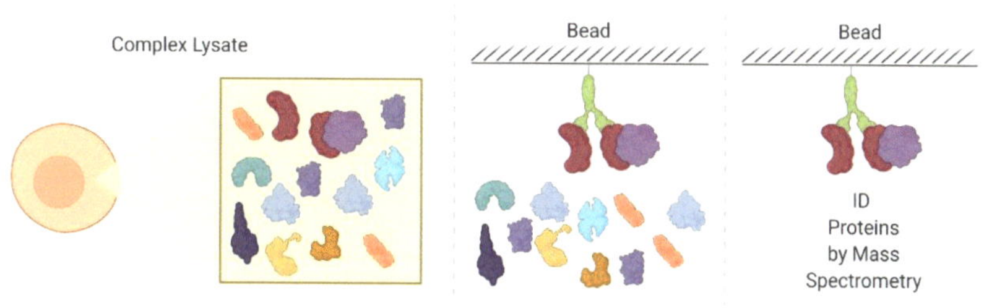

Figure 3.
Affinity purification isolates a protein and any stably interacting protein from a complex solution such as a cell or tissue lysate. Shown here is the most common implementation where an antibody is used to isolate the target protein, followed by unbiased identification of binding proteins using MS. the antibody is attached to a solid substrate to allow for physical manipulations of the target protein.

Approach	Readout
AP-MS	Mass spectrometry
LUMIER	Luciferase activity
XL-MS	Mass spectrometry

Table 2.
Affinity purification techniques covered in this section. These approaches differ primarily in their readout method.

by the BioPlex project, have driven the development of a systematic pipeline that enables high-throughput AP/MS. Such efforts have already resulted in an interaction network with nearly 120,000 interactions identified for over 14,000 proteins in HEK293 cells [18].

A second and more recently developed method is the luminescence-based mammalian interactome mapping (LUMIER). In this approach, a library of epitope-tagged (specifically FLAG-tagged) constructs are co-transfected with a target-of-interest fused to Renilla luciferase. An anti-FLAG antibody is then used to pull down the tagged protein and binding is assayed by reading out luciferase activity of the immunoprecipitate [19]. Though in principle this approach offers increased sensitivity, this technique requires that both the target-of-interest and the library are tagged and expressed using artificial constructs. Thus, the applicability of this method for unbiased screening greatly depends on the accessibility to large libraries of tagged constructs.

While these approaches excel at identifying soluble interactions, ePPIs struggle to survive the processing steps and are noticeably underrepresented in both the LUMIER and even the much more comprehensive BioPlex dataset. One way to address some of the challenges associated to ePPIs is to combine affinity purification with cross-linking, turning transient ePPIs into permanent covalent linkages. By using cross-linking in combination with mass spectrometry (XL-MS), ePPIs can be identified in an unbiased manner. While cross-linking stabilizes weak interactions, XL-MS still has associated challenges like the presence of unproductive cross-links or combinatorial database search space. To overcome these, newly developed cross-linkers used for XL-MS can include affinity tags or MS cleavable moieties [20]. However, these increase cross-linker size and the chances of cross-linking nearby, non-interacting proteins. Existing cross-linking reagents also primarily target reactive amines, limiting the number of protein interactions that can be captured. Cross-linking protein complexes also tends make them less soluble [21]. This is worsened by the fact that ePPIs often involve membrane proteins which already present solubility challenges that complicates down-stream processing. Since extracellular proteins are often heterogeneously post-translationally modified [22], they can be challenging to identify in mass databases for MS experiment. Overall, XL-MS represents one of the few techniques that does not have a bias against ePPIs over soluble PPIs.

While most cross-linking approaches select for general features of proteins like reactive amine groups, alternative strategies have been developed that specifically target cell-surface receptors using trifunctional cross-linkers. These methods typically have one moiety that covalently attaches the cross-linker to the target protein-of-interest, a soluble protein that ranges from peptides, to antibodies or even complex entities such as viral particles. A second moiety links to glycosylated receptor proteins bound to or near the target, and a third moiety enables purification. Three molecules and associated workflows have been described: TRICEPS [23], followed by ASB [24] and HATRIC [25]. These approaches have the potential to enable unbiased study of targets of diverse nature in physiologically relevant settings such as cells expressing endogenous receptors, thus offering an attractive option for ePPI discovery.

2.3 Protein-fragment complementation

2.3.1 Concept description

Protein-fragment complementation refers to methods where a protein with reporter activity is split in two and fused to two proteins being tested for binding. Since the two halves do not interact with each other on their own, reporter activity is only recovered when the halves are fused to interacting proteins. The archetypal example of this approach is the yeast two-hybrid system (Y2H) which uses two halves of a transcriptional factor that can drive the expression of a report gene (**Figure 4**).

2.3.2 Concept pros

Protein-fragment complementation is usually performed using living cells allowing proteins to be maintained in relatively native conditions. Reporter activity often have an amplification step that allows for the sensitive detection of even weak interactions [26]. While protein-fragment complementation technically reads out proximity, reasonable linker lengths can select for small distances. The interaction has to persist long enough for the activity to be reconstituted, reducing false positives rates when compared to some other proximity-based techniques.

2.3.3 Concept cons

Protein-fragment complementation mandates the tagging of proteins with non-native sequences for the reporter readout. These tags can be substantial in size and affect the behavior of the proteins being tagged. Since the reporter activity depends only on the reporter portion being in close proximity, this approach does not guarantee a direct interaction. Most systems only test binary interactions by design since only the tagged proteins are being assayed.

2.3.4 Specific applications

Y2H has been used extensively to detect PPIs since its conception (**Table 3**). The use of yeast allows for low-cost high-throughput testing of interactions. This technique has now been used to detect interactions between 90% of human proteins [27]. However, Y2H is not suited for ePPI discovery. The expression of human proteins in yeast may result in non-native post-translational

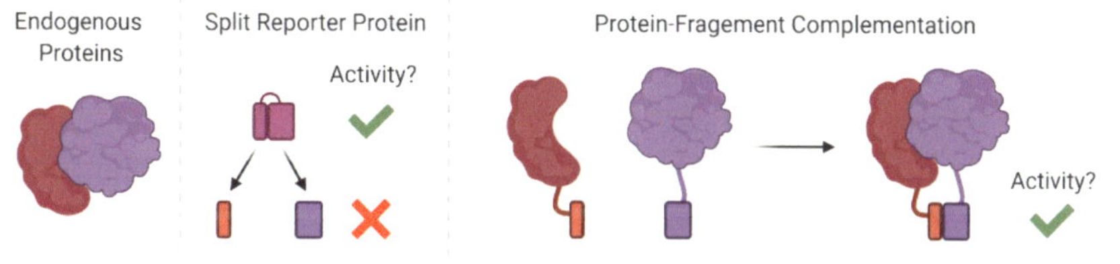

Figure 4.
General schematic for the protein-fragment complementation approach. Two proteins suspected of interaction are each tagged with half of a split reporter protein. The reporter activity is detected only if the split reporter is brought together by an interaction between the two tagged proteins.

Approach	Split reporter system
Yeast two-hybrid	Split Gal4 transcription factor driving reporter expression
MYTH/MaMTH	Split ubiquitin restricting localization of a transcription factor

Table 3.
Specific protein-fragment complementation approaches covered in this section. These differ primarily in the specifics of the split reporter activity.

modifications relevant for function, but more importantly, Y2H actively selects against ePPIs because the interaction must occur in the nucleus to drive transcriptional readout.

To complement the classic Y2H approaches and overcome the pitfalls related to ePPIs, several systems specifically targeting membrane proteins have been developed. The membrane yeast two-hybrid (MYTH) [28] and its mammalian counterpart, mammalian membrane two-hybrid (MaMTH) [29] require that at least one protein being tested is anchored to the plasma membrane. Both of these approaches use a split ubiquitin system where one of the two halves is fused to a membrane protein and a transcription factor. Tethering the transcription factor to the membrane protein keeps it out of the nucleus, preventing reporter expression. When the membrane protein interacts with a protein containing the second half of ubiquitin, a cleavage event occurs, releasing the transcription factor to translocate to the nucleus and initiate reporter expression. In combination with targeted libraries, this approach has been used for the high-throughput detection of interactions between receptor tyrosine kinases and phosphatases [30]. However, since these techniques rely on the endogenous ubiquitin machinery for cleavage, they mandate that both binding partners be expressed in the same cells, limiting applicability of these techniques for detection of in-trans interactors.

2.4 Proximity labeling

2.4.1 Concept description

Proximity labeling techniques identify possible PPIs by covalently modifying proteins that are in close proximity, typically within a few nanometers. In most cases, the label includes an affinity tag like biotin which allows the labeled proteins to be purified and identified using MS (**Figure 5**).

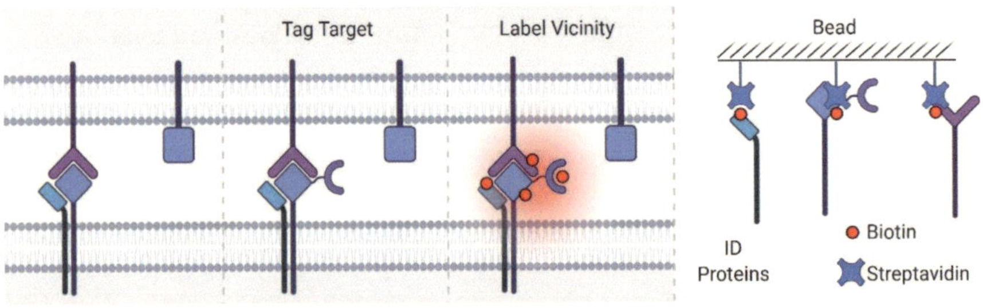

Figure 5.
General schematic of a proximity labeling experiment. A target-of-interest is fused to an enzyme that labels nearby proteins with an affinity tag. That tag can then be used to isolate the proteins for identification.

2.4.2 Concept pros

The different proximity proteomics methods have represented some of the most significant advances in the field of PPI detection, and in particular membrane protein interaction discovery. From the initial development of BioID and its further iterations in BioID2 and TurboID, as well as the more recently developed MicroMap, these techniques have substantially increased the sensitivity for detection of a range of interactions, including weak, transient interactions by translating them into permanent covalent linkages. In addition, proximity proteomics approaches are generally applicable to complex physiological systems and cellular models of interest, and can bypass over-expression of proteins-of-interest and laborious libraries. Furthermore, these approaches also offer the advantage of temporal control, though currently this is typically on the tens of minutes time-scale.

2.4.3 Concept cons

While proximity labeling typically does not require any special equipment, the unbiased identification of proximal proteins requires access to MS. Since these approaches fundamentally readout proximity, the PPI is inferred. Especially if used in complex physiological contexts, the possibility of identifying neighboring but not directly interacting proteins means that this approach has the greatest challenge when it comes to data interpretability. Additionally, the most popular proximity proteomics methods, BioID and APEX, require expression of the protein-of-interest fused to a bulky tag, followed by over-expression of the fusion protein. Although generally applicable to physiologically relevant systems, experimental conditions may require optimization to ensure that the overall behavior of the target-of-interest is not altered by tagging or over-expression.

Currently, these techniques have been applied primarily to detect interactions between proteins on the same cells. In many cases, the utility for in-trans interactions remains to be demonstrated.

2.4.4 Specific applications

The different proximity labeling techniques vary based on what enzymes or chemistries are used to accomplish the labeling. The field of proximity proteomics has been predominantly driven by the development of enzyme-catalyzed proximity labeling. These typically used a promiscuous biotin ligase (from BioID to the much faster TurboID) or a peroxidase (usually APEX or horse radish peroxidase (HRP)) to create a highly reactive biotin species that can only diffuse a short distance before reacting with nearby proteins or water [31]. When a target protein is tagged with one of these enzymes and substrate added, proteins in its vicinity are biotinylated, allowing them to be isolated and identified using MS. The particular techniques differ slightly in their tradeoffs. The peroxidases tend to be more broadly reactive and requiring less labeling time. However, they require the addition of a biotin conjugate and hydrogen peroxide, both of which could be toxic to cells. While the biotin ligases do not have this problem, they are on average slower, though the more recently engineered TurboID can achieve efficient labeling within minutes (**Table 4**) [31].

This concept has been incorporated into specific techniques for identifying ePPIs like selective proteomic proximity labeling assay using tyramine (SPPLAT). SPPLAT uses an HRP-conjugated antibody recognizing a cell surface protein.

Approach	Substrate/Cross-linker Moieties
Biotin ligases (BioID, TurboID)	Biotin
Peroxidases (APEX, HRP)	Different biotin conjugates
SPPLAT	Tyramide biotin conjugates
EMARS	Aryl azide biotin conjugates
MicroMap	Diazirine biotin conjugates

Table 4.
Specific approaches mentioned in this section for using proximity labeling and cross-linking. These techniques differ in the labeling enzymes that they use (for labeling) or the chemistries of the substrate.

Since the antibody cannot diffuse across the plasma membrane, it specifically targets ePPIs without any tagging of proteins, and thus enabling studies in unmodified cellular settings [32]. Another approach is enzyme-mediated activation of radical sources (EMARS) which also uses an HRP-conjugated antibody. However, EMARS uses a biotin fused to an aryl azide group giving it a large labeling radius of 200–300 nm, making it more suitable for characterizing entire microdomains rather than ePPIs [33]. Though the use of antibodies has advantages, genetically tagging a protein with HRP can allow these types of techniques to be performed in the physiological context in an organism. For example, the use of a CD2-HRP fusion protein with a membrane-impermeable biotin-phenol allowed the identification of cell-type specific neural protein cross talk in the fly brain [34].

The newest addition to the proximity labeling family is MicroMap, which uses entirely orthogonal chemistry to the existing techniques. MicroMap uses an antibody to detect the target-of-interest, which is then recognized by a secondary antibody conjugated to a photocatalyst. The photocatalyst absorbs blue light to catalyze the activation of a biotin conjugate molecule in its vicinity. This approach uses a more reactive chemical moiety than the biotin ligase or peroxide approaches, which allow for an even smaller radius of labeling and thus, is more likely to detect direct PPIs. Using MicroMap, the authors proposed a new set of putative binders partners for key immune receptors such as PD-L1 [35].

2.5 Direct protein–protein interaction screens

2.5.1 Concept description

Direct interaction screens encompass a wide variety of techniques that have several features in common. First, there is a query protein that is the target-of-interest. Second, the query protein is tested for binding to a library containing possible binding partners presented as recombinant proteins or receptors expressed on cells. Third, a positive signal in the screen directly reads out an interaction between the query and a given binding partner in the library, using detection methods that vary depending on the approach. Major distinguishing factors between the various direct PPI-screening techniques include: the level of multimerization of the target protein (from monomers to oligomeric proteins), the form of the library of binding partners being screened (protein-based vs. cell-based formats), as well as the degree of purification required (purified protein vs. conditioned media) (**Figure 6**).

2.5.2 Concept pros

This approach typically allows for the opportunity to control most aspects of the screen such as protein concentration and buffer conditions. This approach is also

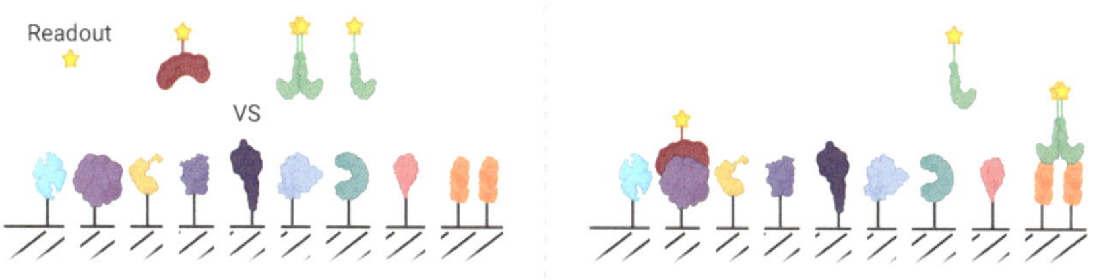

Figure 6.
General schematic for direction protein interactions screens. The library of proteins can be directly immobilized on a solid substrate or be expressed on cells. Alternative multimerization methods have been developed to present the query protein of interest, reviewed in the text.

generally amenable to scale-up. Therefore many modern libraries have high coverage of at least specific protein families. The simplicity and the fact that the readout reflects direct PPIs also generally leads to straight-forward data analysis.

2.5.3 Concept cons

Many of these approaches use purified proteins and may require the use of ectodomains rather than the full-length protein. While the ectodomain is sufficient for binding in many instances, this requirement makes it difficult to identify ePPIs that use multiple ectodomains or transmembrane domains for binding; a behavior documented for the family of seven-transmembrane-domain-containing G protein-coupled receptors (GPCRs). These approaches also typically require that the target-of-interest be screened against a library, which needs to be comprehensive for truly unbiased identification if ePPIs. The generation and maintenance of a large library, either as recombinant proteins or plasmids for expression on cells, can be costly and may require access to automation.

2.5.4 Specific applications

While published work tends to take advantage of specific combinations of the type of target presentation and the type of library, significant mixing and matching is possible due to the similarity in the overall conceptual framework. Therefore, we will talk about the major types of target presentation and library separately and mention any incompatibilities. Also, since there are a large diversity of library formats, we divided the formats into protein-based libraries and cell-based libraries, though the same target presentation strategies can be used for both (**Table 5**).

Target Presentation	Protein-based Library	Cell-based Library
Dimer (Fc tag)	Protein microarray (on slide)	cDNA libraries (on slide)
Pentamer (COMP tag)	Purified protein (in plate)	cDNA libraries (on plate)
Beads-based Multimer (variable)	Purified protein (SPR chip)	CRISPRa gRNA libraries
	Purified protein (Magneto-sensor chip)	Knock-down or Knock-out libraries
	Conditioned media protein (in plate)	

Table 5.
Lists of target presentations and protein and cell-based library formats covered in this section.

2.5.4.1 Target presentation methods

To be able to directly assay interactions, targets-of-interests are typically presented as recombinant protein for this type of approach. While secreted proteins are soluble and can be directly screened, membrane proteins tend to misfold and aggregate if they are extracted from membranes because of their hydrophobic transmembrane domains [12, 13]. Since ectodomains are usually the portion of transmembrane proteins available for direct ePPIs, typically only ectodomains are used for direct ePPI screening.

A number of multimerization approaches that increase query protein avidity and therefore facilitate detection of transient interactions have been developed. In particular, there are three dominant strategies: dimerization induced by fusing ectodomains to the constant Fc region of antibodies [36], pentamerization induced by fusing ectodomains to the rat cartilage oligomeric matrix protein (COMP) [37] and higher order multimerization using small beads with high protein-binding capacity, usually in the form of protein A-coated or streptavidin-coated beads.

While increased multimerization is a major factor for increasing sensitivity with target presentation, the readout method to measure target binding also varies. Using Fc-tagged dimers allows the detection of the target using a variety of secondary antibodies or protein A/G that bind to Fc regions with high affinity [36]. However, using enzymatic readouts can add a high degree of signal amplification that allows for increased sensitivity. Therefore, the approach used to generate the largest ePPI networks to date uses pentamerization combined with an enzymatic β-lactamase colorimetric assay [37–40]. As for bead-based approaches, the specific readout can be magnetic, fluorescent or chemiluminescent depending on the specific screening method used [41, 42].

Lastly, some of the recent high-throughput technologies use conditioned media enriched for the target-of-interest rather than purified proteins. Using conditioned media involves direct capture of secreted protein or protein ectodomains in the absence of protein purification, thus minimizing potential inactivation of the proteins due to purification steps. The use of conditioned media can also save time and resources, helping to make the approaches more accessible to different laboratory and more amenable to scaling up [37–40].

2.5.4.2 Protein-based library formats

Different protein-based library formats can allow for different levels of throughput and information collected about the binding interactions. The most common and high-throughput approaches are generally qualitative, detecting whether the interaction is present, but not providing quantitative information such as kinetic parameters. One example of this type of library is the protein microarray, which for ePPIs, contains different purified secreted proteins or ectodomains directly spotted on slides. Only small amounts of each protein are used, allowing for the dense tiling of thousands of proteins per slide. The compact format allows slides to be covered with a small volume of fluorescently-labeled target protein, rinsed and imaged using microscopy [43]. While this is a convenient format, the construction of the protein microarrays is often costly because it requires all of the proteins to be purified.

Another type of library for qualitative ePPI identification uses plate-based screening formats. The use of plates allows for the easy addition of proteins and controlled washes without the need for specialized microfluidics. While purified proteins can be used, plate-based formats allow for the direct capture of secreted tagged proteins from conditioned media. Capture of biotinylated proteins using streptavidin-coated plates [37] or Fc-tagged proteins using Protein A-coated plates [38–40] followed by washing allows for the effective purification of library proteins in wells while adding sensitivity by multimerizing (in the case of multivalent binding of streptavidin to biotin) or capturing already multimerized proteins. This approach also allows the use of enzymatic liquid phase readouts: β-lactamase-based colorimetric assays or luciferase-based luminescence assays which provides an additional degree of signal amplification. The plate-based approach also gives one value per well, allowing for simple data analysis and the greatest interpretability.

While the plate-based approach is generally the most scalable options, other techniques trade some scale for quantitative information on ePPIs. In particular, microfluidics, automation and miniaturization has pushed label-free biophysical techniques to be more high-throughput. For example, the combination of microfluidics and either surface plasmon resonance (SPR) or magneto-nanosensors has increase the scale enough to study all combinatorial interactions between a small number of proteins, making it especially adept at addressing complex cross-talk between small interaction networks [44, 45]. While SPR is the gold standard technique for biophysical characterization of protein interactions and calculation of kinetic parameters, the magneto-nanosensor platform provides higher degrees of sensitivity, and therefore, requiring less material to detect weak ePPIs. However, it requires the use of magnetic nanoparticles conjugated to the target-of-interest. The nanoparticles are are flowed over patches of library proteins printed on magneto-nanosensors that detect a change in electrical resistance if a nanoparticle is nearby [45]. Another technique that also provides similar information is biolayer interferometry (BLI) which translates protein binding into a light interference signal. While typically less sensitive than SPR and the magneto-nanosensor platform, BLI excels in its ease-of-use. BLI uses small, disposable sensors that can be coupled to targets-of-interest, typically through the capture of tag like Fc-tags or biotin. The sensors are then simply dipped into wells containing the potential binding partners in solution. With advances in automated and miniaturized BLI setups, it can be used to screen for interactions in high-throughput, provided that libraries of recombinant proteins are available. This technology helped identify the PVR-TIGIT interaction [46] which is mechanistic foundations of the anti-TIGIT immunotherapy [47].

2.5.4.3 Cell-based library formats

Even though protein-based libraries have many advantages such as storability and easy data interpretation, they can often fail to detect ePPIs because of biochemical challenges associated with membrane proteins. Many membrane proteins lose activity when truncated into soluble ectodomains or extracted from membranes. In addition, the complex cellular membrane environment can provide important protein and non-protein co-factors, orient and cluster membrane proteins and assist in high-order complex formation. Therefore, hard to purify receptors are often screened against cDNA libraries expressing membrane proteins directly on cells. This is especially true for important drug targets like GPCRs and ion channels [48] which have multiple transmembrane domains and typically small extracellular regions.

To screen for interactions using cell-based formats, libraries are used to either induce loss-of-function (lack of binding) or gain-of-function (increased binding). In the loss-of-function approach, possible binders of a target-of-interest are knocked down or knocked out either randomly using chemical mutagens or transposons like gene trap [49] or in a targeted manner with siRNA, zinc-finger nuclease, transcription activator-like effector nuclease (TALEN) or clustered regularly interspaced short palindromic repeat (CRISPR) libraries [50]. When the target-of-interest is incubated with the cells, the target should not interact if the interaction partner has been depleted. However, it may be difficult to identify cells that bind the target-of-interest. In addition, the interaction must to be simple enough that knocking down one interaction partner causes a detectable decrease in binding.

To avoid these limitations, an alternative approach is to overexpress receptors that may participate in ePPIs. This is most commonly done using cDNA libraries. The DNA libraries are spotted on slides [51] or plated into wells [52], with each spot or well containing a vector encoding for a different protein. Cells are then added and transfected to induce them to overexpress the protein and display them on the plasma membrane. If the cells are expressing the receptor for the target-of-interest, this can be detected by increased target binding to the surface of the cell. This approach has been successfully utilized to deorphanize secreted factors [53], interactions between immune receptors [54], or identify glycan-dependent recognition of specific ligands [55]. However, the generation and management of cDNA libraries that have significant coverage of membrane proteins can be expensive and not accessible to many investigators. In addition, selective expression of the myriad of possible receptors isoforms that may participate in ligand binding makes truly comprehensive cDNA libraries infeasible. One way to address isoform-specific expression while facilitating library management is to use CRISPR activation (CRISPRa). In this implementation, CRISPR-Cas9 fused to transcriptional activation domains is coupled to guide RNAs selectively targeting cell-surface genes to overexpress receptor proteins. A high coverage CRISPRa guide library targeting most cell surface proteins has been recently utilized to identify novel receptor-ligand interactions [56].

2.6 Computational models

2.6.1 Concept description

Computational models cover a large range of concepts that attempt to predict PPIs based on existing knowledge of the biochemistry of protein binding and features of proteins, such as the sequence, conserved residues or structural features.

2.6.2 Concept pros

Computational models can offer relatively less resource-consuming and faster alternatives to experimental research. They allow for the theoretical exploration of PPIs without regard for experimental challenges related to expression of proteins or development of workflows or platforms. Modern machine learning approaches may also identify unintuitive features that are the most predictive for interactions such as unappreciated modifications. They can also draw from larger pools of information, taking into account protein expression patterns, genetic variations and dysregulation in disease.

2.6.3 Concept cons

Computational modeling approaches to identify PPIs, not to mention ePPIs, are still in their infancy, with overall low rates of accuracy. Many are based on our existing knowledge of experimentally determined interactions, which may have biases and is incomplete. Approaches that attempt to model binding interfaces are too computationally expensive to be high-throughput even when experimentally determined protein structures exist [57].

2.6.4 Specific applications

Since computational approaches remain immature for human ePPIs, we will mostly highlight the different computational resources and a few different

Approach	Details
STRING	Database of PPIs predictions based on public data
BioGRID	Database of curated public PPI data
BioPlex	Database of human PPI identified by AP/MS
Coevolution	PPI prediction based on coevolution of residues
PICTree	Functional clustering using hidden Markov models
FpClass	PPI prediction using machine learning

Table 6.
List of computational resources and approaches covered in this section.

approaches rather than try to describe a list of the major algorithms. However, this is a rapidly developing area mirroring the explosion in available experimental datasets, including data from all of the approaches mentioned so far as well as expression data for cell types, tissue and now single cells identifying which proteins are at the same places at the same times (**Table 6**) [58, 59].

The increased availability of comprehensive databases for PPIs, and more recently ePPIs, have fueled diverse computational approaches. Efforts like STRING [60] and BioGRID [61] which collects and curates public data on PPIs, are often drawn on for model development and are also important resources for individual researchers looking for the next interaction to drug. There are also many databases that document the progress of specific approaches like BioPlex which contains thousands of human interactions identified by AP/MS [18] as well as the Research Collaboratory for Structural Bioinformatics Protein Data Bank which captures many structures showing the molecular details of PPIs [62]. However, even here ePPIs have posed a challenge because we do not have a definitive list of all proteins that reach the cell surface in various tissues and cell types, though ongoing efforts are trying to experimentally answer that question [59, 63–65]. Recently, the human surfaceome was estimated using a machine learning model to predict the cell surface localization of almost 3000 proteins [66].

Modeling approaches that actually attempt to predict ePPIs range in terms of the types of information they try to account for. While not yet applied to human ePPIs, the use of residue-residue coevolution in combination with structure modeling successfully predicted many ePPIs in bacteria [67]. Another approach, PICTree, focused on the structurally related immunoglobulin superfamily (IgSF) of proteins, using knowledge of family members with known binding partners and sequence conservation to predict new interactions using [68]. Lastly, some approaches use broad information sets about a gold standard set of interactions. For example, FpClass trains their model on everything amino acid makeup to post-translational modifications to expression patterns [69]. However, this still resulted in an estimated false discovery rate of 60%, which shows that while modeling can assist in hypothesis generation, there is more work to be done before modeling would take the place of experimental approaches.

3. Summary

Extracellular protein–protein interactions are an important set of possible drug targets. They are commonly dysregulated in disease and can be targeted to alter disease phenotypes. Practically, ePPIs are exposed on the cell surface, making them easier to access using therapeutic approaches. However, because of challenges associated with ePPI biochemistry, most membrane proteins and secreted factors do not have identified interactions. Elucidating the extracellular interaction networks in humans as well as their dysregulation during disease will be key to understand basic biology and fuel new or improved drug development efforts. To tackle this daunting challenge, researchers have applied genetic, chemical, biochemical and computational approaches to come up with an ever-growing list of ePPIs. Here we have reviewed the progress made in the last decade in technologies suitable for the study of ePPIs. In particular, we discuss those approaches that can be applied to the high throughput screening of ePPIs in an unbiased fashion.

4. Future perspectives

As costs are continually falling on readouts like sequencing and mass spectrometry, and as throughput increases with better automation and computational analysis, the future looks bright in the field of ePPI identification. More and more techniques will cross over the categories that we have laid out, finding middle points that balance the various tradeoffs of ease, interpretability, and physiological relevance.

One exciting development that 2020 brought was the release of two large-scale efforts using ePPI-optimized pentamer-based direct interaction screening approaches. These efforts each systematically tested hundreds of thousands of pairwise interactions, focusing on the IgSF of single-pass transmembrane proteins, the largest family of secreted and membrane-expressed proteins in the human genome [39, 40]. These large interaction networks identified hundreds of new interactions and present the most extensive ePPI network maps to date.

Once the interactions are found, we need to be able to manipulate them in humans to cure diseases. While not the topic of this chapter, several exciting developments on the drug development front holds much promise for targeting ePPIs. New highly selective inhibitors that recognize the transmembrane domains of protein, such as the isoform-selective inhibitor of the Nav1.7 channel, can provide novel classes of chemical inhibitors of transmembrane proteins to disrupt ePPIs [70]. While cytokines often offer desirable ways to manipulate many immune functions, they are often like playing with fire because of their many disparate effects. However, with improvements in protein design, completely artificial cytokine mimics can now be made which can be highly selective for activities that are desired and counter selected for activities that are not [71].

One major challenge that lies ahead is to not to just identify ePPIs but to identify disease relevant human ePPIs. Along these lines, a recently published map of the IgSF highlighted the power of big data integration, showing that the combination of clinical data with a focus on the protein pair participating in ePPIs gave greater predictive value than each of the proteins alone [39], suggesting that targeting specific ePPIs may be more beneficial than targeting an individual protein. Another challenge is the reliance on animal models. Plasma membrane and secreted factors are some of the least conserved of all proteins [72], having to evolve to adapt to our unique physiology. As more complex human ePPI networks are discovered, it will be a challenge to understand their impacts at the organismal level. Whether it be organoid systems or better functional assays, with the rapid growth in ePPI identification technologies, soon we'll have to find high-throughput ways to ask, what do they do?

5. Executive summary

- Extracellular protein–protein interactions (ePPIs) make for good drug targets because they control many biological processes and are accessible to therapeutic agents.

- An estimated third of all human genes encode for proteins that may be involved in ePPIs, necessitating high-throughput approaches for unbiased discovery.
- General PPI detection techniques often fail to overcome challenges posed by extracellular proteins, leading to the development of ePPI-specific approaches.
- EPPI-specific technologies address some of these challenges directly, such as using multimerization to strengthen characteristically weak interactions or assaying interactions on cells to avoid difficult membrane protein purifications.
- Techniques typically balance several tradeoffs, mainly: control and interpretability versus physiological relevance, rates of false positive versus false negative results, and scale and coverage versus time and expense.
- Specific techniques fall into broad categories: biochemical fractionation, affinity purification, protein-fragment complementation, proximity labeling, direct interaction and computational modeling that can be synergistic for ePPI discovery.
- New ePPIs are still being discovered with the aid of new techniques, suggesting that many remain to be found. The methodologies discussed in this chapter should set the bases for identification and characterization of novel ePPIs in humans and other model organisms.

Acknowledgements

We thank Genentech Reviewers for critically reading the manuscript. Figures were created with BioRender.com. **Figure 1A** was adapted from "Tumor Microenvironment" and **Figure 1B** was adapted from "Proposed Therapeutic Treatments for COVID-19 Targeting Viral Entry Mechanism", by BioRender.com (2020). Retrieved from https://app.biorender.com/biorender-templates

Conflict of interest

Both authors are Genentech employees and own shares in the Roche/Genentech group.

Author details

Shengya Cao and Nadia Martinez-Martin*
Genentech, South San Francisco, CA, USA

*Address all correspondence to: nadia.martinez@almirall.com

References

[1] WHO|Projections of mortality and causes of death, 2016 to 2060. [cited 2020 Nov 18]. Available from: https://www.who.int/healthinfo/global_burden_disease/projections/en/

[2] Libby P, Ridker PM, Maseri A. Inflammation and atherosclerosis. Circulation. 2002;105(9):1135-1143.

[3] Vinay DS, Ryan EP, Pawelec G, Talib WH, Stagg J, Elkord E, et al. Immune evasion in cancer: Mechanistic basis and therapeutic strategies. Semin Cancer Biol. 2015;35:S185–S198.

[4] Mayor R, Carmona-Fontaine C. Keeping in touch with contact inhibition of locomotion. Vol. 20, Trends in Cell Biology. 2010. p. 319-28.

[5] Carmeliet P, Jain RK. Angiogenesis in cancer and other diseases. Nature. 2000 Sep;407(6801):249-257.

[6] Abercrombie M. Contact inhibition and malignancy. Nature. 1979 Sep;281(5729):259-262.

[7] Hoffmann M, Kleine-Weber H, Schroeder S, Krüger N, Herrler T, Erichsen S, et al. SARS-CoV-2 Cell Entry Depends on ACE2 and TMPRSS2 and Is Blocked by a Clinically Proven Protease Inhibitor. Cell. 2020;181(2):271-280.e8.

[8] Shang J, Wan Y, Luo C, Ye G, Geng Q, Auerbach A, et al. Cell entry mechanisms of SARS-CoV-2. Proc Natl Acad Sci U S A. 2020;117(21).

[9] Marchio P, Guerra-Ojeda S, Vila JM, Aldasoro M, Victor VM, Mauricio MD. Targeting early atherosclerosis: A focus on oxidative stress and inflammation. Oxid Med Cell Longev. 2019;2019(Ldl).

[10] Hegde PS, Chen DS. Top 10 Challenges in Cancer Immunotherapy. Immunity. 2020;52(1):17-35.

[11] Hansen J, Baum A, Pascal KE, Russo V, Giordano S, Wloga E, et al. Studies in humanized mice and convalescent humans yield a SARS-CoV-2 antibody cocktail. Science (80-). 2020;369(6506):1010-4.

[12] Wright GJ, Martin S, Bushell KM, Söllner C. High-throughput identification of transient extracellular protein interactions. Biochem Soc Trans. 2010;38(4):919-922.

[13] Martinez-Martin N. Technologies for proteome-wide discovery of extracellular host-pathogen interactions. J Immunol Res. 2017;2017.

[14] Oppenheim JJ. Cytokines: Past, present, and future. Int J Hematol. 2001;74(1):3-8.

[15] Havugimana PC, Hart GT, Nepusz T, Yang H, Turinsky AL, Li Z, et al. A census of human soluble protein complexes. Cell. 2012;150(5):1068-1081.

[16] Depner H, Lützkendorf J, Babkir HA, Sigrist SJ, Holt MG. Differential centrifugation-based biochemical fractionation of the Drosophila adult CNS. Nat Protoc. 2014;9(12):2796-2808.

[17] Owald D, Khorramshahi O, Gupta VK, Banovic D, Depner H, Fouquet W, et al. Cooperation of Syd-1 with Neurexin synchronizes pre-with postsynaptic assembly. Nat Neurosci. 2012;15(9):1219-1226.

[18] Huttlin EL, Bruckner RJ, Navarrete-Perea J, Cannon JR, Baltier K, Gebreab F, et al. Dual Proteome-scale Networks Reveal Cell-specific Remodeling of the Human Interactome. bioRxiv. 2020;2020.01.19.905109. Available from: https://www.biorxiv.org/content/biorxiv/early/2020/01/19/2020.01.19.905109.full.pdf

[19] Barrios-Rodiles M, Brown KR, Ozdamar B, Bose R, Liu Z, Donovan RS, et al. High-throughput mapping of a dynamic signaling network in mammalian cells. Science (80-). 2005;307(5715):1621-5.

[20] Chavez JD, Mohr JP, Mathay M, Zhong X, Keller A, Bruce JE. Systems structural biology measurements by in vivo cross-linking with mass spectrometry. Nat Protoc. 2019;14(8): 2318-2343.

[21] Iacobucci C, Götze M, Sinz A. Cross-linking/mass spectrometry to get a closer view on protein interaction networks. Curr Opin Biotechnol. 2020;63:48-53.

[22] Kolarich D, Jensen PH, Altmann F, Packer NH. Determination of site-specific glycan heterogeneity on glycoproteins. Nat Protoc. 2012;7(7): 1285-1298.

[23] Frei AP, Jeon OY, Kilcher S, Moest H, Henning LM, Jost C, et al. Direct identification of ligand-receptor interactions on living cells and tissues. Nat Biotechnol. 2012;30(10):997-1001.

[24] Tremblay TL, Hill JJ. Biotin-Transfer from a trifunctional crosslinker for identification of cell surface receptors of soluble protein ligands. Sci Rep. 2017;7(December 2016):1-9.

[25] Sobotzki N, Schafroth MA, Rudnicka A, Koetemann A, Marty F, Goetze S, et al. HATRIC-based identification of receptors for orphan ligands. Nat Commun. 2018;9(1):1-8.

[26] Estojak J, Brent R, Golemis EA. Correlation of two-hybrid affinity data with in vitro measurements. Mol Cell Biol. 1995;15(10):5820-5829.

[27] Luck K, Kim DK, Lambourne L, Spirohn K, Begg BE, Bian W, et al. A reference map of the human binary protein interactome. Nature. 2020;580(7803):402-408.

[28] Stagljar I, Korostensky C, Johnsson N, Te Heesen S. A genetic system based on split-ubiquitin for the analysis of interactions between membrane proteins in vivo. Proc Natl Acad Sci U S A. 1998;95(9):5187-5192.

[29] Petschnigg J, Groisman B, Kotlyar M, Taipale M, Zheng Y, Kurat CF, et al. The mammalian-membrane two-hybrid assay (MaMTH) for probing membrane-protein interactions in human cells. Nat Methods. 2014;11(5):585-592.

[30] Yao Z, Darowski K, St-Denis N, Wong V, Offensperger F, Villedieu A, et al. A Global Analysis of the Receptor Tyrosine Kinase-Protein Phosphatase Interactome. Mol Cell. 2017;65(2): 347-360.

[31] Branon TC, Bosch JA, Sanchez AD, Udeshi ND, Svinkina T, Carr SA, et al. Efficient proximity labeling in living cells and organisms with TurboID. Nat Biotechnol. 2018;36(9):880-898.

[32] Rees JS, Li XW, Perrett S, Lilley KS, Jackson AP. Selective proteomic proximity labeling assay using tyramide (SPPLAT): A quantitative method for the proteomic analysis of localized membrane-bound protein clusters. Curr Protoc Protein Sci. 2015;2015(April): 19.27.1-19.27.18.

[33] Honke K, Kotani N. Dentification of cell-surface molecular interactions under living conditions by using the enzyme-mediated activation of radical sources (EMARS) method. Sensors (Switzerland). 2012;12(12): 16037-16045.

[34] Li J, Han S, Li H, Udeshi ND, Svinkina T, Mani DR, et al. Cell-Surface Proteomic Profiling in the Fly Brain Uncovers Wiring Regulators. Cell. 2020;180(2):373-386.e15.

[35] Geri JB, Oakley J V, Reyes-Robles T, Wang T, McCarver SJ, White CH, et al. Microenvironment mapping via Dexter energy transfer on immune cells. Science. 2020;367(6482):1091-1097.

[36] Czajkowsky DM, Hu J, Shao Z, Pleass RJ. Fc-fusion proteins: New developments and future perspectives. EMBO Mol Med. 2012;4(10):1015-1028.

[37] Bushell KM, Söllner C, Schuster-Boeckler B, Bateman A, Wright GJ. Large-scale screening for novel low-affinity extracellular protein interactions. Genome Res. 2008;18(4): 622-630.

[38] Martinez-martin N, Marcandalli J, Huang CS, Lanzavecchia A, Perez L, Martinez-martin N, et al. An Unbiased Screen for Human Cytomegalovirus Identifies Neuropilin-2 as a Central Viral Receptor Article An Unbiased Screen for Human Cytomegalovirus Identifies Neuropilin-2 as a Central Viral Receptor. Cell. 2018;174(5):1158-1171.e19.

[39] Verschueren E, Husain B, Yuen K, Sun Y, Paduchuri S, Senbabaoglu Y, et al. The Immunoglobulin Superfamily Receptome Defines Cancer-Relevant Networks Associated with Clinical Outcome. Cell. 2020;182(2): 329-344.e19.

[40] Wojtowicz WM, Vielmetter J, Fernandes RA, Siepe DH, Eastman CL, Chisholm GB, et al. A Human IgSF Cell-Surface Interactome Reveals a Complex Network of Protein-Protein Interactions. Cell. 2020;182(4):1027-1043.e17.

[41] Bosse R, Illy C, Chelsky D. Principles of AlphaScreen, Amplified Luminescent Proximity Homogenous Assay. Appl Note. :1-8.

[42] Husain B, Ramani SR, Chiang E, Lehoux I, Paduchuri S, Arena TA, et al. A platform for extracellular interactome discovery identifies novel functional binding partners for the immune receptors B7-H3/CD276 and PVR/CD155. Mol Cell Proteomics. 2019;18(11):2310-2323.

[43] Zhu H, Bilgin M, Bangham R, Hall D, Casamayor A, Bertone P, et al. Global analysis of protein activities using proteome chips. Science (80-). 2001;293(5537):2101-5.

[44] Piliarik M, Vaisocherová H, Homola J. A new surface plasmon resonance sensor for high-throughput screening applications. Biosens Bioelectron. 2005;20(10 SPEC. ISS.):2104-10.

[45] Lee JR, Bechstein DJB, Ooi CC, Patel A, Gaster RS, Ng E, et al. Magneto-nanosensor platform for probing low-affinity protein-protein interactions and identification of a low-affinity PD-L1/PD-L2 interaction. Nat Commun. 2016;7:1-9.

[46] Yu X, Harden K, Gonzalez LC, Francesco M, Chiang E, Irving B, et al. The surface protein TIGIT suppresses T cell activation by promoting the generation of mature immunoregulatory dendritic cells. Nat Immunol. 2009;10(1):48-57.

[47] Johnston RJ, Comps-Agrar L, Hackney J, Yu X, Huseni M, Yang Y, et al. The Immunoreceptor TIGIT Regulates Antitumor and Antiviral CD8+ T Cell Effector Function. Cancer Cell. 2014;26(6):923-937.

[48] Santos R, Ursu O, Gaulton A, Bento AP, Donadi RS, Bologa CG, et al. A comprehensive map of molecular drug targets. Nat Rev Drug Discov. 2016;16(1):19-34.

[49] Carette JE, Guimaraes CP, Varadarajan M, Park AS, Wuethrich I, Godarova A, et al. Haploid genetic screens in human cells identify host factors used by pathogens. Science (80-). 2009;326(5957):1231-5.

[50] Fernández A, Josa S, Montoliu L. A history of genome editing in mammals. Mamm Genome. 2017;28(7-8):237-246.

[51] Freeth J, Soden J. New Advances in Cell Microarray Technology to Expand Applications in Target Deconvolution and Off-Target Screening. SLAS Discov. 2020;25(2):223-230.

[52] Wood L, Wright GJ. High-Content Imaging for Large-Scale Detection of Low-Affinity Extracellular Protein Interactions. SLAS Discov. 2019;24(10): 987-999.

[53] Mullican SE, Lin-Schmidt X, Chin CN, Chavez JA, Furman JL, Armstrong AA, et al. GFRAL is the receptor for GDF15 and the ligand promotes weight loss in mice and nonhuman primates. Nat Med. 2017;23(10):1150-1157.

[54] Bhatt RS, Berjis A, Konge JC, Mahoney KM, Klee AN, Freeman SS, et al. KIR3DL3 is an inhibitory receptor for HHLA2 that mediates an alternative immunoinhibitory pathway to PD1. Cancer Immunol Res. 2020;canimm. 0315.2020.

[55] Sun Y, Senger K, Baginski TK, Mazloom A, Chinn Y, Pantua H, et al. Evolutionarily conserved paired immunoglobulin-like receptor α (PILRα) domain mediates its interaction with diverse sialylated ligands. J Biol Chem. 2012;287(19):15837-15850.

[56] Chong ZS, Ohnishi S, Yusa K, Wright GJ. Pooled extracellular receptor-ligand interaction screening using CRISPR activation. Genome Biol. 2018;19(1):1-16.

[57] Macalino SJY, Basith S, Clavio NAB, Chang H, Kang S, Choi S. Evolution of in silico strategies for protein-protein interaction drug discovery. Molecules. 2018;23(8).

[58] Petryszak R, Keays M, Tang YA, Fonseca NA, Barrera E, Burdett T, et al. Expression Atlas update - An integrated database of gene and protein expression in humans, animals and plants. Nucleic Acids Res. 2016;44(D1):D746–D752.

[59] Thul PJ, Lindskog C. The human protein atlas: A spatial map of the human proteome. Protein Sci. 2018;27(1):233-244.

[60] Szklarczyk D, Gable AL, Lyon D, Junge A, Wyder S, Huerta-Cepas J, et al. STRING v11: Protein-protein association networks with increased coverage, supporting functional discovery in genome-wide experimental datasets. Nucleic Acids Res. 2019;47(D1):D607–D613.

[61] Oughtred R, Stark C, Breitkreutz BJ, Rust J, Boucher L, Chang C, et al. The BioGRID interaction database: 2019 update. Nucleic Acids Res. 2019;47(D1): D529–D541.

[62] Burley SK, Berman HM, Bhikadiya C, Bi C, Chen L, Di Costanzo L, et al. RCSB Protein Data Bank: Biological macromolecular structures enabling research and education in fundamental biology, biomedicine, biotechnology and energy. Nucleic Acids Res. 2019;47(D1): D464–D474.

[63] Bausch-Fluck D, Hofmann A, Bock T, Frei AP, Cerciello F, Jacobs A, et al. A mass spectrometric-derived cell surface protein atlas. PLoS One. 2015;10(4):1-22.

[64] Regev A, Teichmann SA, Lander ES, Amit I, Benoist C, Birney E, et al. The Human Cell Atlas. Elife. 2017 Dec 5;6:1-31.

[65] Roberts B, Haupt A, Tucker A, Grancharova T, Arakaki J, Fuqua MA, et al. Systematic gene tagging using CRISPR/Cas9 in human stem cells to

illuminate cell organization. Mol Biol Cell. 2017;28(21):2854-2874.

[66] Bausch-Fluck D, Goldmann U, Müller S, van Oostrum M, Müller M, Schubert OT, et al. The in silico human surfaceome. Proc Natl Acad Sci. 2018;201808790.

[67] Cong Q, Anishchenko I, Ovchinnikov S, Baker D. Protein interaction networks revealed by proteome cocvolution. Science (80-). 2019;365(6449):185-9.

[68] Yap EH, Rosche T, Almo S, Fiser A. Functional clustering of immunoglobulin superfamily proteins with protein-protein interaction information calibrated hidden markov model sequence profiles. J Mol Biol. 2014;426(4):945-961.

[69] Braun P, Tasan M, Dreze M, Barrios-Rodiles M, Lemmens I, Yu H, et al. An experimentally derived confidence score for binary protein-protein interactions. Nat Methods. 2009;6(1):91-97.

[70] Ahuja S, Mukund S, Deng L, Khakh K, Chang E, Ho H, et al. Structural basis of Nav1.7 inhibition by an isoform-selective small-molecule antagonist. Science (80-). 2015;350(6267).

[71] Silva DA, Yu S, Ulge UY, Spangler JB, Jude KM, Labão-Almeida C, et al. De novo design of potent and selective mimics of IL-2 and IL-15. Nature. 2019;565(7738):186-191.

[72] Ramilowski JA, Goldberg T, Harshbarger J, Kloppman E, Lizio M, Satagopam VP, et al. A draft network of ligand-receptor-mediated multicellular signalling in human. Nat Commun. 2015;6.

Chapter 4

Design and Implementation of High Throughput Screening Assays for Drug Discoveries

Fawzi Faisal Bokhari and Ashwag Albukhari

Abstract

The process of drug discovery is challenging and a costly affair. It takes about 12 to 15 years and costs over $1 billion dollars to develop a new drug and introduce the finished product in the market. With the increase in diseases, virus spread, and patients, it has become essential to invent new medicines. Consequently, today researchers are becoming interested in inventing new medicines faster by adopting higher throughput screening methods. One avenue of approach to discovering drugs faster is the High-Throughput Screening (HTS) method, which has gained a lot of attention in the previous few years. Today, High-Throughput Screening (HTS) has become a standard method for discovering drugs in various pharmaceutical industries. This review focuses on the advancement of technologies in High-Throughput Screening (HTS) methods, namely fluorescence resonance energy transfer (FRET), biochemical assay, fluorescence polarization (FP), homogeneous time resolved fluorescence (HTRF), Fluorescence correlation spectroscopy (FCS), Fluorescence intensity distribution analysis (FIDA), Nuclear magnetic resonance (NMR), and research advances in three major technology areas including miniaturization, automation and robotics, and artificial intelligence, which promises to help speed up the discovery of medicines and its development process.

Keywords: Drug discovery and development, High-Throughput Screening, fluorescence resonance energy transfer, biochemical assay, fluorescence polarization (FP), homogeneous time resolved fluorescence (HTRF), Fluorescence correlation spectroscopy (FCS), Fluorescence intensity distribution analysis (FIDA), Nuclear magnetic resonance (NMR), miniaturization, automation and robotics, and artificial intelligence

1. Introduction

It takes about 12 to 15 years and costs over $1 billion dollars to develop a new drug and introduce the finished product in the market. Moreover, the process is highly complex and costly as huge investments are made into technology [1, 2]. There is a need to reduce costs, increase efficiency and introduce drugs conveniently and faster to the market by higher throughput methods. The High-throughput screening method screens millions of chemical and biological compounds in a short interval of time. It is an automated process and screens many biological or chemical compounds for their therapeutic potential. The

High-throughput screening method efficiently accelerates the discovery of drugs, which are of potentially great therapeutic promise compared with other screening methods [3–5].

This review highlights the types of High-throughput screening assays and different detection techniques such as fluorescence resonance energy transfer (FRET), biochemical assay, fluorescence polarization (FP), homogeneous time resolved fluorescence (HTRF), Fluorescence correlation spectroscopy (FCS), Fluorescence intensity distribution analysis (FIDA) [6], Nuclear magnetic resonance (NMR), and research advances in three major technology areas including miniaturization, automation and robotics, and artificial intelligence, which has shown great promise to speed the discovery of medicines and its development process [7, 8].

1.1 Understanding high-throughput screening process for the discovery of drugs

In the high-throughput screening process, many compounds are screened to find potential candidate compounds that efficiently affect a biological target. These so-called candidate compounds are referred to as 'hits.' As an example, the high-throughput screening process successfully identified a potent pan-SRC kinase inhibitor now known as 'Dasatinib, BMS-354825' for the biological target of diabetes. The high-throughput screening processes involve various detection methods such as robotics or plate readers and corresponding software to process and analyze the data obtained. Once the 'hits' are discovered, further analysis in the high-throughput screening process can enable one to understand the potential optimization of the 'hits' achieved during the first screening round [9–11].

It is essential to understand that the high-throughput screening method alone cannot wholly evaluate a potential drug as toxicity studies are further needed for this evaluation. Instead, high-throughput screening is essential to eliminate the time that would have been wasted on investigating compounds that had little or no desired effect on the biological target. Through the utilization of this automated screening process, millions of compounds can together be screened and compounds with no or poor effects eliminated [10].

Basically, in the process of high-throughput screening HTS high number of effectors and biological modulators are screened and assayed against specific and selected targets. The high-throughput screening HTS process ensures that the time taken to screen large compound libraries is reduced and the whole drug discovery process is speeded up. In this manner, the high-throughput screening HTS method can be capable of screening more than thousand compounds per day [12]. It is ideally a mechanism-based approach where compounds are screened to provide improved drugs. High-throughput screening process precisely focuses on single mechanism contributing to identification of target specific compounds. The high-throughput screening HTS assays helps to screen various types of libraries such as genomics, protein, combinatorial chemistry, and peptide libraries [10]. The high-throughput screening HTS and assay method includes various steps such as preparation of reagents, target identification, compound management, assay development, and high throughput library screening, which are performed with extreme care and precision. The detail steps are as follows [13].

Firstly, targets are selected. There are presently around 500 targets that are being utilized by various companies. Among these targets, cell membranes receptors, mostly G-protein coupled receptors are commonly used and comprise the largest group with 45% of the total, followed by Enzymes (28%), hormones (11%), unknowns (7%), ion-channels (5%), nuclear receptors (2%), and DNA (2%). Off late pharmaceutical companies are interested to analyze compounds that interfere or modulate the function of GPCRs [13].

Undoubtedly, the integration of different compound libraries with wide chemical diversity in the high throughput screening method is a potential solution for massive drug discovery. The identification of good hits via the high throughput screening method can effectively reduce the time frame of discovering drugs in the process. However, for the screening technique to be successful various factors are dependent on it. Various factors that are essential to be considered are quality and number of validated targets, diversity and number of compounds, and the capability to screen compounds in a cost effective and timely manner using robust informative assays. Not just that, there are certain limitations of the high throughput screening method that defines the pharmacological properties of active compounds such as, synthetic chemistry for lead optimization and the low throughput of secondary assays. This major drawback causes a major hindrance to the overall identification rate of potential candidates for clinical evaluation. Due to this reason, researchers and scientists are trying to develop better technological solutions to overcome these challenges.

1.2 Application of high throughput screening (HTS) in drug discoveries

Applications of High-throughput screening (HTS) method in drug discoveries are detailed below

1.3 In screening

- For screening of novel biological active compounds
- Various natural products
- Combinatorial libraries such as peptides, chemicals etc.
- Biological libraries
- RNA chips
- DNA chips
- Protein chips

Generally, High-throughput screening process is carried pout via a microliter plate. Today, modern micro plates for HTS assays are performed in automation-friendly microliter plates with a 96, 384, 1536 or 3456 well format. The so called wells successfully comprise of experimentally useful matter, often an aqueous solution of dimethyl sulfoxide (DMSO) and some other chemical compound, the latter of which is different in each well across the plate [14].

Today, in most of the drug discovery labs, the collection of libraries has increased from 400,000 to more than 1 million compounds. In order to screen these high numbers of compound libraries automated 384 wells or higher density single compound test formats are used. Ideally, the primary screen is responsible and designed for rapid identification of hits from this library of compounds. The aim is to achieve a minimum number of false positives and maximum number of confirmed hits. Not to mention, the hit rates generally range between 0.1 – 5%, depending on the assay. The hit range or number also depends on the cutoff parameters that are set by the researchers, or the dynamic range of a given assay. These Primary screens run in multiples of single compound concentrations. The results of the primary screening method are expressed in terms of percent activity as a negative (0 percent) and a positive (100 percent) control. The achieved Hits are further retested, generally independently from the first assay. After retesting, if a compound displays the same activities, it is accepted as a confirmed hit, and the process go through secondary screening or lead optimization. The results obtained from the secondary screening method are used to decide and further filter the substances that will make it on to clinical trials [13].

The combination of screening methods with bioinformatics, allows potential drugs to be efficiently and quickly screened, and hence discovering drugs at a faster speed and, which can be explored in more detail. The Initial screening of these compounds for their binding ability is the main role of high-throughput screening method. The high-throughput screening process generally involves developing tests, or assays, where in the potential compounds are made to bind with proteins, causing visible change that can be automatically read by a sensor. Generally, this change is achieved by light emissions by a fluorophore in the reaction mixture. The way the process works out is that, fluorophores are attached to target proteins in such a way that its ability to fluoresce is diminished (quenched) when the protein binds to another molecule. Then a different system measures the difference in polarization, which is a property of light, emitted by unbound versus bound fluorophores. Usually, bound fluorophores are highly polarized and hence can be easily detected by sensors. Various detection technologies for high throughput s screening are available today these includes time-resolved fluorescence (TR-FRET), fluorescence resonance energy transfer (FRET), fluorescence polarization, luminescence and absorbance. Not to mention these methods required efficient, highly sensitive, and versatile multi-mode micro plate readers [13].

Generally, libraries are referred as sets of compounds produced by combinatorial chemistry. Depending on how the solid-phase are handled, these compounds may be either mixtures or individual compounds. In biological assays range of compounds present in the libraries are tested as follows.

- Test of mixture in solutions
- Test of individual compounds in solutions
- Test of compounds on the beads

1.4 Test of mixture in solutions

In this test method the compounds are cleaved from the beads and tested in solution. Sometimes, it is a tedious task to find the compounds that are active by observing the pharmacological screen. In order to carry out successful identification of the most active compounds, it is essential to resynthesize the componenets individually. In this manner the process of screening and resynthesizing in an iterative manner is one of the most successful and simple methods for the identification of most potent components from libraries.

1.5 Test of individual compounds in solutions

A second method of testing compounds is the separation of the beads manually into individual wells and cleaving the compounds from the solid-phase. These compounds are then tested as individual entities.

Method	Traditional Screening	High – Throughput Screening
Assay Format	Single Tube	Array Format 96-Well
Assay Volume	~1 ml	50-100 µl
Compound Used	~5-10 mg	~1 µg
Assay Compounds	Added Singly	Added Simultaneously
Mechanical Action	1:1	1:96
Compound/Solution	Dry/Custom Solution	In Solution/DMSO
Assay Speed	Slow & Laborious	Fast and Efficient (~1 min/step/96-well plate)
Screening Ability	20-50 Compounds/Week/Lab	1000-10,000 Week/Lab
Diversity Screening	Limited Number	Unlimited Number

Table 1.
Based on 96 well format.

1.6 Test compounds on the beads

Another method for screening is testing on the beads. This is carried out by the application of fluorescent assay or colorimetric technique. In this process appropriate beads can be chosen by fluorescence or color, and picked out by micromanipulation. Further the the product structure of the active compounds, if a peptide, can be determined by sequencing on the bead. Whereas, non-peptide structures can be identified by one of the tagging methods.

1.7 Applications

High-throughput technology finds wide applications in areas other than drug development. These include the following

- Genomics
- Protein Analysis
- DNA Sequencing

1.8 Traditional screening vs. high-throughput

Traditional methods were time consuming as compared to high-throughput discovery. The table below demonstrates the differences between traditional methods and high-throughput methods. As shown in **Table 1**, screening ability of high-throughput screening ability increased 50 times on the low end, and 200 times on the high end as compared to traditional screening [3]. Leading to an increase of efficacy and accuracy, in High-throughput screening method. Moreover in high-throughput screening method minimal amounts of test compounds are used [12].

2. Types of high throughput assays

Assays are segregated into cell-based assays and biochemical assays. Biochemical assays are further segregated into homogeneous and heterogeneous assays [15].

2.1 Homogeneous assay

Homogeneous assay measurement is a single step process, where reagents are added in a single stage or multiple steps. Steps involved are fluid addition, incubation and readings. The homogeneous assay measurement is characterized by the interaction between the surrounding environment and the analyte. The homogeneous assay measurement method can be coupled with different detection techniques such as fluorescence, radiometric etc. for HTS. The advantageous feature of the homogeneous assay measurement method is that it is simple and involves minimum steps thereby contributing to reduce cost and minimum robotic complexity required in automation. One of the drawback of the homogeneous assay measurement method is that there are interference in measurements as it is carried out in the presence of other assay components and having a signal to background ratio of less than 10 [15].

2.2 Heterogeneous assays

Heterogeneous assays measurement method is a bit more complicated than the homogeneous assay method as it involves a few additional steps such as filtration, centrifugation etc. These additional steps ensures that the component(s) to be measured are separated from rest of the components, which may cause interference in assays measurement method and hence contributing to high signal to background ratio. A thumb rule always followed is that when homogeneous assay fails or high signal to background ratio is required, heterogeneous assay measurement method is generally carried out [15].

2.3 Biochemical assays

Biochemical assays are protein, enzyme-based, or receptor assays that utilizes a designated target in a more purified form. Generally speaking, biochemical assays are frequently carried out using scintillation proximity assay (SPA), radiometric, colorimetric fluorescence detection techniques. In the Scintillation Proximity Assay technology binding reactions are assayed without carrying out the filtration or washing process step. In this technique radioactive labels emitting electrons at about 10 μm in water are used to carry out the assay. Generally, SPA technique is a preferred method for all surface cell receptors when high binding and low receptor density is required [15].

One of the biochemical assays technique is Fluorescence resonance energy transfer. This technique is further summarized in the next sections [15].

2.4 Fluorescence resonance energy transfer (FRET)

FRET technique is a non-radiative quantum mechanical process, where energy is transferred from an excited donor fluorophore to a suitable acceptor fluorophore. Here, energy from incident light is absorbed onto the donor fluorophore and it is transferred to nearby acceptor molecule [15].

There are certain conditions that must be fulfilled for an effective FRET assay:

i. Ensuring effective overlap between the donor molecules fluorescence emission spectrum and the acceptor chromophore's excitation or absorption spectrum. The degree of overlap is termed as spectral overlap integral (J).

ii. The acceptor and donor fluorophore must be as close to each other (typically 1-10 nanometer).

iii. Ensuring significant difference in the extent of quenching of the starting material and product.

iv. Ensuring that the transition dipole orientations of the acceptor and donor are almost parallel. (SANGEETA SAINI, Syed Arshad Hussain)

v. Limitation of Fluorescence resonance energy transfer technique FRET:

vi. It needs an external illumination for the initiation of fluorescence transfer to occur.

vii. Possibility of direct excitation of the acceptor or to photo-bleaching. To avoid this, Bioluminescence Resonance Energy Transfer technique (or **BRET**) is used, which uses a bioluminescent luciferase from sea pansy *Renillaren iformis*to produce an intialpoton [15].

2.5 Fluorescence polarization (FP)

The Fluorescence polarization technique is widely used in high throughput screening method. In this technique when light is irradiated to the fluorophore, it gets excited and emits light in same polarized plane. The fluorophore remains steady throughout the excitation state. However, if the fluorophore changes its position i.e., it rotates during excitation state, it emits light in different plane (depolarized). Larger molecule tends to show little movement while smaller molecule rotates quickly and giving high and low polarization value [15, 16].

2.6 Applications

i. The Fluorescence polarization technique has been used in ligand/receptor studies, Tyrosine Kinase Assays etc.

ii. The Fluorescence polarization technique has also successfully found application in quantifying biochemical properties such as attachment of proteins to nucleic acid, protein denaturation etc. [15].

2.7 Homogeneous time resolved fluorescence (HTRF)

The HTRF method is a combination of time resolved measurement (TR) of fluorescence and standard FRET technology, thereby allowing the elimination of short-lived background Fluorescence, which occurs due to interfering materials in the sample and allowing a delay of approximately 50 to 150μseconds between the initial excitation and fluorescence measurement. Homogeneous time resolved fluorescence method utilizes europium cry ptate (Eu3 + cryptate) as fluorescent energy donor, which are rare earth complexes consisting of a macrocycle within which a Eu3+ ion is tightly embedded. This cage behaves as an antenna, collecting and transferring energies to the Eu3+ ion that eventually releases this energy with a specific long lived fluorescent pattern. Cryptate comprise of cross-linked allophycocyanin or XL665, a phycobilli protein pigment purified from red algae as acceptor [15].

In a recent research study HTRF was used as a screening application for the assay of tyrosine kinase and screening against tumor necrosis factor receptor in a 384-well microplate.. It was observed that (HTRF) was similar and related to fluorescence intensity techniques. The detector was gated for a short time period of

(10 ns) - > and the initial burst of fluorescence was not measured. Post this gating period the longer lasting fluorescence of the sample was measured. HTRF is effectively used to enhance sensitivity levels [15].

Applications of HTRF and FRET methods:

- In studies of molecular interaction and immunoassays.
- There exist many reagents pre-labeled with HTRF donors, which can be adapted to many assays.

2.8 Fluorescence correlation spectroscopy (FCS)

FCS is a confocal fluorescence where parameters of prime importance are the fluctuation of the fluorescence intensity, occurring from noise as well as biological, chemical, and physical effects on the fluorophore. Changes in chemical and physical properties, like equilibria, reactions, complexation, quenching, and like molecular motion, photophysical interactions, changes in conformation affects the overall emission [15].

2.9 Applications

1. Enabling the determination of various molecular interactions.
2. Enabling the study of conformation changes.
3. Enabling efficient diffusion analysis by concentration and aggregation measurements.
4. Enabling applications in binding assays and enzymatic assays.
5. Enabling structural and molecular dynamics of fluorescent proteins in vivo and in vitro.

2.10 Fluorescence intensity distribution analysis (FIDA)

The FIDA technique involves the monitoring of the sample's fluorescence intensity with a heterogeneous brightness profile. Hence, it help to determine the concentrations and specific brightness values of a number of individual fluorescent species in a solution [15].

2.11 Nuclear magnetic resonance (NMR)

Nuclear magnetic resonance based screening is an effective method to help identify leads of low molecular weight organic compound which bind to the protein targets. The screening method provides information on the binding location and affinity of potential lead compounds. This method is especially useful in the designing of highly selective lead structures or when hallow binding pockets need to be targeted. However, the technique is extremely sensitive toward loose fragment binders offering comparatively high throughput.

This Nuclear magnetic resonance NMR based screening method not only provides information of the binding site or the conformation of the bound ligand but it also reveals information related with docking of the ligand to the protein's binding pocket [15].

3. Cell based assays

Cell-based assays in HTS method are classified under following classes: [6].

3.1 Second messenger assays

The Second messenger assays are used to efficiently measure fast, transient fluorescent signals occurring in matter of seconds or milliseconds. It monitors signal transduction from activated cell-surface receptors. Many fluorescent molecules are known to respond to changes in intracellular.

Calcium ion concentration, membrane potential and various other parameters, hence they are The second messenger assays are made of fluorescent molecules as these molecules are known to respond to changes in intracellular Calcium ion concentration, membrane potential, and various other parameters, So, the fluorescent molecules are used in second messenger assays for receptor stimulation and ion-channel activation. The development of hydrophobic voltage-sensitive probes and FRET-compatible microplate instrumentation has helped the advancement of the screening technique for ionchannel drug discovery [15].

3.2 Reporter gene assays

The reporter gene assays monitors cellular responses at translation levels. It is responsible for indicating the absence or presence of gene products and in turn reflecting changes in a signal transduction pathway. The quantifications of reporters are generally performed by various bio-chemical methods i.e., by measuring enzymatic activities. Typically, plasmids are used as reporter genes [15].

3.3 Cell proliferation assays

Cell proliferation assays are responsible for monitoring the overall growth or no growth responses of the cell to external stimuli. Cell proliferation assays can be quickly and easily employed for automation [15].

3.4 Statistics

It is essential to achieve quality hits with high degree of confidence in drug discovery process. Errors occur or issues arise when analytical method for hit selection is repeated under similar conditions. In real case scenarios obtained results differ from each other and there occurs variability in the system under studies. Using statistical tools in analyzing screening experiments is the correct approach for the interpretation of screening data, and hence supporting making right decisions [15].

4. Breakthrough technologies

4.1 Automation and robotics

In the high-throughput screening process, large numbers of samples are screened, microplates having up to 3456 wells are generally used to hold the samples. Primarily, automation plays an essential role in the high-throughput screening process enabling millions of compounds to be rapidly screened in shorter time periods, as opposed to laboratory benchtop investigation of compounds by researchers in the same period [2, 17].

However, there are various challenges faced in automation. For instance, the reagents quantity added to each well of a microplate has to be minimized in order for the potential compounds screening experiment to be designed within the constraints presented by automation. Other challenges include limiting the adjustments that can be made to compounds through the screening process. The means that only one single injection of compound is applicable to target samples. Hence, further adjustments cannot be made to how compounds are added to samples as the experimental design is would no longer be suitable for automation process [2].

Automation is generally categorized into three common modes namely, batch, semi-automated, and integrated. These three modes differ in functions such as walk away capabilities, flexibility, complexity and numbers of tasks. For example, in the batch mode, scientist still need to load stacks of plates, which are further limited to fewer steps in the process. On the other hand, Integrated automation, is a more sophisticated process, which is capable out of performing multiple scheduled steps facilitated by a robotic mover, further allowing non-manual operation for long periods [2, 18].

Often the automated solution requires the operator to be well skilled with the automation process. If not so, specialized training are provided from the equipment. Batch automation are often performed with little specialized training of the operators. Today automation has evolved and become more democratized as compared to the scenario ten years ago. This trend reduces the need for specialized training of the operators in the future and further making such solutions commercially available [2].

A further process involved in high-throughput screening is a robotic configuration. Often a robotic system is incorporated into high-throughput screening platforms to accelerate the time by which data is acquired [2].

The system essentially would be able to perform multiple functions such as adding reagents, transferring microplates, mixing samples, and incubating samples at specific temperatures. This enables both experimental times to be reduced and the elimination of any error that could potentially be brought about if the process was carried out manually [2].

4.2 Miniaturization

Today researchers aim to reduce the cost the process even more than current high-throughput screening technology. Miniaturization is a technology where smaller or lesser sample quantities are utilized to provide results, in the aim to reduce cost of using more samples. However, smaller quantities must provide reliable results. Development in miniaturization introduces higher sensitivity microplates for high-throughput screening, which can reliably measure signals from small sample sizes and overcoming the challenges of the initial miniaturization technology [2].

However, it is predicted that in the further miniaturization of the screening process can be achieved in future, thus reducing costs of the process even more than current high-throughput screening technology [2].

Most of the steps in HTS lead discovery are influenced by miniaturization. First step in miniaturization is increasing the density of plate well to more than a 96-well standard. Target densities of about 384, 1536, and 3854 wells per plate are available. Hence, higher throughput screening (HTS) achieved through this method of miniaturization majorly reduces the reagent costs as reaction volumes decreases from 10 to 20 mL in the well of a 384-well plate down to <2 mL in the well of a 1536-well plate [2, 19].

It is quite challenging to handle fluids in miniaturized assays, nevertheless it is a crucial parameter for performance. It is difficult to dispense compounds that are stored or solubilized in organic solvents, in a fast, controllable, and accurate manner. Additional issues include effective mixing, clogging, and evaporation that need to be resolved. Ebner states that "One of the most common problems that high-throughput labs have to address is spatial or edge effects." When poor cellular growth occurs at the perimeter of the wells as compared to growth of the cells in the rest of the plate, the phenomena is called as edge effect. As a consequence, these challenges tend to restrict the plate density to about 384-wells. Microfluidic technology, is a more extreme form of miniaturization, helps to addresses some of these known fluid handling challenges. Microfluidic chips replaces the liquid handling mechanics with channels connected to liquid reservoirs while providing the benefits of reduced volumes. In most cases, the devices comprise of integrated tools including electrodes built-in and combines multiple operational steps [7, 20].

Microfluidic devices are also capable of isolating single cellsthat can be further cultured on the chips. This ability of microfluidic devices eliminates cellular heterogeneity on cancer cell populations as an example. Traditional drug screening methods see response information from an average of all cells. The microfluidic solution allows analysis of a single cell's antidrug response. In addition to this cell-on-chip model, recent advances have led to tissue-on-chip and organ-on-chip models which are still early in development [21]. Someday, these chip models may provide an alternative to animal models [22]. Because they are early in development, they are not high- throughput solutions today. But they show great promise to speed determination of drug activity, optimal combinatorial drug screening and toxicity testing in the future [2].

4.3 Artificial intelligence

Artificial intelligence (AI) has found great applications in medicinal chemistry for designing compounds and the discovery of drugs since the 1960s. A well-known Machine-learning tool like quantitative structure–activity relationship modeling has played a very important role to help in the identification of various useful target molecules from millions of compounds. Today, the application of Artificial intelligence has expanded onto drug discovery and tasks including image analysis, robotics control, and logistics. Artificial intelligence has also expanded its application in the process of drug discoveries namely hit identification, target selection, lead optimization, efficiently helping in preclinical and clinical trial studies [2, 23–25].

New applications of Artificial intelligence in drug discovery process now lets the researchers and scientists supervise the system as opposed to driving the system manually. Moreover, Artificial intelligence combined with robotic systems provides automation of the design, build, test, and learn (DBTL) cycle, resulting in a system for designing experiments, executing it, data analysis, hence, the optimization and execution of experiments iteratively. Consequently the application of artificial intelligence decreases the number of experiments to be performed and helps to generate the best possible optimization. In practice such systems have been developed and demonstrated at the University of Illinois. The new fully-automated system outperformed traditional screening methods by 77% and evaluated less than 1% of possible variants [2, 26].

Following are the advantageous features of Artificial intelligence in drug discovery applications [2, 4].

i. Helps in cutting down of the time by more than half to develop a potential drug candidate from lead molecule.

ii. Predicted molecules by Artificial intelligence are Helpprecise.

iii. No time is wasted on testing irrelevant molecules, as compared to traditional methods that test 90% of the irrelevant molecules [27].

iv. Currently, Artificial intelligence is capable of discovering novel compounds that are more selective and potent. This is achieved by quicker speed of high quality screening data sets at an affordable cost as compared to the expensive and slower screening method alone.

An area where artificial intelligence plays an essential role is the field of personalized or "precision" medicine [28]. Precision medicines are basically growing drugs in the industry. In the development process of personalized medicine collections of healthy and diseased human samples are needed [4]. Usually, the samples are sequenced using next-generation sequencing technique, resulting in the generation of massive data. The application of Artificial intelligence and methods of deep learning helps in the efficient analysis of big data sets [25].

5. Conclusions

The primary goal of high-throughput screening processes is to screen through a library of compounds, and help in the identification of candidates that affect the target in a desired way. This phenomena is referred as "hits" or "leads". Generally, hits are achieved by using various technologies including liquid handling devices, plate readers, robotics, and software for data processing. Today automation and robotics has been widely accepted in the drug discovery process and great progress continues to be made in this area. Automated process provides better process consistency and hence, better data quality. Alternatively, automation not only allows scientists to walk away freely and pursue other tasks, but it also allows trail of traceability if any questions arise. The process of automation minimizes human errors [29].

To sum it up, HTS processes does not particularly helps in the identification of drugs, because HTS cannot assess several properties that are critical for developing new drug. For example, HTS method cannot evaluate properties like bioavailability and toxicity. Instead, the primary role of HTS assays is to help in the identification of "leads" and provide suggestions for their optimization. Hence, the results from HTS assays helps to reveal the initial point for further steps in the drug discovery process, including drug design. HTS assays also helps to understand the interaction or role of a particular biochemical process.

Hence, the HTS method should be accepted as a technology that scans biological library quickly and efficiently excluding compounds showing no effect in the analysis. Various academic institutions and mainly industries use high-throughput screening method to screen large number of compounds on a daily basis. Various detection techniques FCS, NMR, HRTF etc., contribute to the screening of compounds in large number.

According to market analysis, the global (HTS) market size was at 15.3 billion USD in 2020 and is projected to reach 26.4 billion USD by 2025, growing at a CAGR of 11.5% in the forecast period. Market growth is driven by factors including improving research and development spent by biotechnological and pharmaceutical companies, advancements in high throughput screening technologies, availability of funding from government, and capital investments from various bodies. As we all are aware of the outbreak of the corona virus, in response to this, various biopharmaceutical, pharmaceutical companies, and small startups have stepped forward to develop solution to this issue. Scientists and researchers were able to find list of molecules that could target COVID-19. As per the latest reports, there are 79 available vaccine candidates, out of which 20 vaccine candidates are in the third stage of clinical trials. Out of the 20 vaccine candidates, eleven of them have been authorized in various countries. Researchers and scientists have taken the initiative to speed drug discovery process by using high throughput screening method and found few promising drugs that can be used against COVID-19 namely Remdesivir, Chloroquine & Hydroxychloroquine, Lopinavir & Ritonavir, and Lopinavir with Ritonavir plus Interferon beta-1a. There has been an increase in drug discovery projects in efforts to treat COVID-19, which is the driving force for the growth of the high-throughput screening products market [30].

Off late, pharmaceutical & biotechnology industries are collaborating with various academic and research institutions to implement drug discovery more efficiently. The industries and the institution works hand in hand as institutions perform target identification and validation of research, while industries carry out high throughput screening assay development and screening campaigns. In this manner the industries and research institutes, benefits from this collaboration [30].

However, there are certain hindrances to the growth of the high throughput screening market. The commercially available assay platforms are applicable for the already established target classes namely G-protein coupled receptors, ion-channels, nucleic acids, and enzymes. However, today there exists addition of target classes such as transmembrane receptors, transporters, signaling pathways, protein–protein interactions, protein-RNA interactions, and protein-DNA interactions leading to numerous complexities (such as protein instability and reagent variability) in the field of assay development & target identification and being a barrier to the growth of the high throughput screening market [30].

Owing to this expansion of new target classes, researchers and scientist must be encouraged to invest their efforts in developing new essay platforms [30].

6. Executive summary

- The chapter highlights the different phenomenal concepts of HTS including fluorescence resonance energy transfer (FRET), biochemical assay, fluorescence polarization (FP), homogeneous time resolved fluorescence (HTRF), Fluorescence correlation spectroscopy (FCS), Fluorescence intensity distribution analysis (FIDA), Nuclear magnetic resonance (NMR).

- The chapter also illustrates the various types of HTS applications.

- A key factor for successful HTS protocols, optimization of precise conditions and environments for the production of optimal "hits".

- HTS is the selected experimental method for drug sensitization by screening thousands of drug compounds offered as libraries in a single day.
- Applications of HTS may include but not limited to, novel drug discoveries, natural products, biological libraries, DNA & RNA chips, and protein chips.
- Screening ability of high-throughput screening ability increased 50 times on the low end, and 200 times on the high end as compared to traditional screening.
- Different assays can be used for end-results such as cell-based assays, second messenger assays, reporter gene assays, and cell proliferation assays.
- Artificial intelligence (AI) has been widely used in HTS for selection of hits and potential targets.

7. Future directions

- HTS for bioactive small molecules can be identified through marine natural products to address ectopic issues.
- Artificial intelligence is coming to be more precise in the identification and selection of hits and potential targets.
- Recent research papers have pave the way for using HTS to identify novel potential small molecule inhibitors that can be used to inhibit bacterial, viral or parasitic replication.
- Recent HTS protocols have highlighted the importance of using HTS in the identification of modulators and activators of important pathways.
- Recent reports of HTS using spheroid 3D gastric carcinoma cells unleash new trends of using 3D cells in high-content imaging.

Author details

Fawzi Faisal Bokhari[1*] and Ashwag Albukhari[2,3]

1 Regional Academic Affairs, Armed Forces Hospitals – Taif Region, Taif, Saudi Arabia

2 Department of Biochemistry, Faculty of Sciences, King Abdul Aziz University, Jeddah, Saudi Arabia

3 Centre of Artificial Intelligence in Precision Medicine, King Abdul Aziz University, Jeddah, Saudi Arabia

*Address all correspondence to: fawzi_bokhari@hotmail.com

References

[1] Ncardia. Fully automated, high-throughput screening for drug discovery [Internet]. Ncardia. 2018. Available from: https://www.ncardia.com/innovations/automated-hts-drug-discovery.html

[2] Brubacher MG. High-throughput Technologies in Drug Discovery [Internet]. Technology networks. 2021. Available from: https://www.technologynetworks.com/drug-discovery/articles/high-throughput-technologies-in-drug-discovery-330193

[3] Dickinson ME, Flenniken AM, Ji X, Teboul L, Wong MD, White JK, et al. High-throughput discovery of novel developmental phenotypes. Nature [Internet]. 2016 Sep 22;537(7621):508-14. Available from: http://www.nature.com/articles/nature19356

[4] Jayshree Pandya. Biobanking Is Changing The World [Internet]. Forbes. 2019 [cited 2021 Apr 19]. Available from: https://www.forbes.com/sites/cognitiveworld/2019/08/12/biobanking-is-changing-the-world/?sh=4c9864473792

[5] Carnero A. High throughput screening in drug discovery. Clin Transl Oncol [Internet]. 2006 Jul;8(7):482-490. Available from: http://link.springer.com/10.1007/s12094-006-0048-2

[6] Silverman L, Campbell R, Broach JR. New assay technologies for high-throughput screening. Curr Opin Chem Biol [Internet]. 1998 Jun;2(3):397-403. Available from: https://linkinghub.elsevier.com/retrieve/pii/S136759319880015X

[7] Brubacher MG. High Throughput Screening for Drug Discovery: Continually Transitioning into New Technology [Internet]. Technology n. technology networks; 2020 [cited 2021 Apr 19]. Available from: https://www.technologynetworks.com/drug-discovery/articles/high-throughput-technologies-in-drug-discovery-330193

[8] Segall M. Smart high-throughput screening. Drug Discov Today [Internet]. 2003 Feb;8(4):160-161. Available from: https://linkinghub.elsevier.com/retrieve/pii/S1359644603025984

[9] Labs B. High Throughput Screening Assays for Drug Discovery [Internet]. Bellbrook Labs. 2021. Available from: https://www.bellbrooklabs.com/high-throughput-screening-assays-drug-discovery/

[10] Chacko AR. Application of High-Throughput Screening in Drug Discovery [Internet]. AZO Life Science. 2021. Available from: https://www.azolifesciences.com/article/Application-of-High-Throughput-Screening-in-Drug-Discovery.aspx

[11] Pusterla T. High-throughput screening (HTS) [Internet]. BMG Lab Tech. 2019. Available from: https://www.bmglabtech.com/high-throughput-screening/

[12] Hosseinzadeh S. Navigating Drug Discovery with High-Throughput Screening [Internet]. High-throughput Discovery. 2021 [cited 2021 Apr 19]. Available from: https://htds.wordpress.ncsu.edu/topics/novel-high-throughput-micro-nanofluidic-technology/

[13] Shukla AA. High Throughput Screening of Small Molecule Library: Procedure, Challenges and Future. J Cancer Prev Curr Res [Internet]. 2016 Jun 15;5(2). Available from: https://medcraveonline.com/JCPCR/high-throughput-screening-of-small-molecule-library-procedure-challenges-and-future.html

[14] Rudd J. High Throughput Screening – Accelerating drug discovery efforts [Internet]. Technology networks. 2017. Available from: https://www.technologynetworks.com/tn/articles/high-throughput-screening-accelerating-drug-discovery-efforts-288926

[15] Hajare AA, Salunkhe SS, Mali SS, Gorde SS, Nadaf SJ, Pishawikar SA. Review on: high-throughput screening is an approach to drug discovery. Am J PharmTech Res [Internet]. 2013;4:112-129. Available from: https://www.academia.edu/download/46793533/Review_on_High-throughput_screening_is_a20160625-20141-4oxox.pdf

[16] Hall MD, Yasgar A, Peryea T, Braisted JC, Jadhav A, Simeonov A, et al. Fluorescence polarization assays in high-throughput screening and drug discovery: a review. Methods Appl Fluoresc [Internet]. 2016 Apr 28;4(2):022001. Available from: https://iopscience.iop.org/article/10.1088/2050-6120/4/2/022001/meta

[17] Cronk D. High-throughput screening. In: Drug Discovery and Development [Internet]. Elsevier; 2013. p. 95-117. Available from: https://linkinghub.elsevier.com/retrieve/pii/B9780702042997000081

[18] Wildey MJ, Haunso A, Tudor M, Webb M, Connick JH. High-throughput screening. Annu Rep Med Chem [Internet]. 2017;50:149-195. Available from: https://www.sciencedirect.com/science/article/pii/S0065774317300076

[19] Dunn DA, Feygin I. Challenges and solutions to ultra-high-throughput screening assay miniaturization: submicroliter fluid handling. Drug Discov Today [Internet]. 2000;5:S84–S91. Available from: https://www.sciencedirect.com/science/article/pii/S1359644600800896

[20] Sun J, Warden AR, Ding X. Recent advances in microfluidics for drug screening. Biomicrofluidics [Internet]. 2019;13(6):61503. Available from: https://scholar.google.com/citations?user=SRXx_eUAAAAJ&hl=en&oi=sra

[21] Dittrich PS, Manz A. Lab-on-a-chip: microfluidics in drug discovery. Nat Rev Drug Discov [Internet]. 2006;5(3):210-218. Available from: https://www.nature.com/articles/nrd1985

[22] Probst C, Schneider S, Loskill P. High-throughput organ-on-a-chip systems: Current status and remaining challenges. Curr Opin Biomed Eng [Internet]. 2018;6:33-41. Available from: https://www.sciencedirect.com/science/article/pii/S2468451117300909

[23] Brubacher MG. High-throughput Technologies in Drug Discovery [Internet]. Technology Networks. 2020. Available from: https://www.technologynetworks.com/drug-discovery/articles/high-throughput-technologies-in-drug-discovery-330193

[24] Sellwood MA, Ahmed M, Segler MH, Brown N. Artificial intelligence in drug discovery. Future Med Chem [Internet]. 2018 Sep;10(17):2025-2028. Available from: https://www.future-science.com/doi/full/10.4155/fmc-2018-0212

[25] Zhang L, Tan J, Han D, Zhu H. From machine learning to deep learning: progress in machine intelligence for rational drug discovery. Drug Discov Today [Internet]. 2017;22(11):1680-1685. Available from: https://www.sciencedirect.com/science/article/pii/S1359644616304366

[26] HamediRad M, Chao R, Weisberg S, Lian J, Sinha S, Zhao H. Towards a fully automated algorithm driven platform for biosystems design. Nat Commun [Internet]. 2019;10(1):1-10. Available from: https://www.nature.com/articles/s41467-019-13189-z

[27] SLAS. AI and Machine Learning Facilitates Faster Path to Personalized Medicine [Internet]. SLAS. 2019 [cited 2021 Apr 19]. Available from: https://www.slas.org/publications/electronic-laboratory-neighborhood/2019-eln-articles/ai-and-machine-learning-facilitates-faster-path-to-personalized-medicine/

[28] Parexel. The Future of Drug Development: The Implementation of Precision Medicine for Successful Oncology Drug Development [Internet]. Pharma voice. 2019 [cited 2021 Apr 19]. Available from: https://www.pharmavoice.com/contributed-article/drug-development-precision-medicine-oncology/

[29] Entzeroth M. Emerging trends in high-throughput screening. Curr Opin Pharmacol [Internet]. 2003 Oct;3(5):522-529. Available from: https://linkinghub.elsevier.com/retrieve/pii/S1471489203000882

[30] MarketsandMarkets. High-Throughput Screening (HTS) Market by Product (Instruments, Software, Service), Technology (Cell-Based Assays, Label-Free), Application (Drug Discovery, Biochemical Screening, Research), End User (Pharma & Biotech, CROs)- Global Forecast to 2025 [Internet]. MarketsandMarkets. 2021 [cited 2021 Apr 19]. Available from: https://www.marketsandmarkets.com/Market-Reports/high-throughput-screening-market-134981950.html

Section 4

High-Throughput Screening Based Cell Signalling Modulators for Novel Drug Designing/Development

Chapter 5

Targeting the Aryl Hydrocarbon Receptor (AhR): A Review of the In-Silico Screening Approaches to Identify AhR Modulators

Farag E.S. Mosa, Ayman O.S. El-Kadi and Khaled Barakat

Abstract

Aryl hydrocarbon receptor (AhR) is a biological sensor that integrates environmental, metabolic, and endogenous signals to control complex cellular responses in physiological and pathophysiological functions. The full-length AhR encompasses various domains, including a bHLH, a PAS A, a PAS B, and transactivation domains. With the exception of the PAS B and transactivation domains, the available 3D structures of AhR revealed structural details of its subdomains interactions as well as its interaction with other protein partners. Towards screening for novel AhR modulators homology modeling was employed to develop AhR-PAS B domain models. These models were validated using molecular dynamics simulations and binding site identification methods. Furthermore, docking of well-known AhR ligands assisted in confirming these binding pockets and discovering critical residues to host these ligands. In this context, virtual screening utilizing both ligand-based and structure-based methods screened large databases of small molecules to identify novel AhR agonists or antagonists and suggest hits from these screens for validation in an experimental biological test. Recently, machine-learning algorithms are being explored as a tool to enhance the screening process of AhR modulators and to minimize the errors associated with structure-based methods. This chapter reviews all *in silico* screening that were focused on identifying AhR modulators and discusses future perspectives towards this goal.

Keywords: human AhR, in silico, in vitro, AhR modulator, crystal structure, AhR modeling

1. Introduction

Six decades ago, researchers made extensive studies to answer a puzzling question. That was how administrating exogenous substances such as polycyclic aromatic hydrocarbons (PAHs) had a potent induction on xenobiotic-metabolizing enzymes in rats' livers [1, 2]. It was finally Alan Poland and his colleagues who finally answered this question in the early 1970s. Poland discovered a novel hepatic protein in complex with the polycyclic aromatic hydrocarbons compound, 2,3,7,8-tetrachlorodibenzo-p-dioxin (TCDD) [2]. The new protein was bound to TCDD in a potent affinity and was isolated from hepatic cytosolic fractions of mice C57BL/6, a mice model strain for studying aromatic hydrocarbon responsiveness.

This protein was later termed as the aryl hydrocarbon receptor (AhR) [2] and was identified as a ligand-activated transcription factor.

Later studies showed that AhR is expressed in several tissues including but not limited to; liver, lung, placenta, and heart and different cell types throughout the developmental periods of organ growth [3]. Further knockout studies in mice revealed essential functions for AhR in multiple physiological and pathophysiological pathways [4–6]. This accumulated knowledge over the last decades defined AhR as an environmental sensor for air pollutants and as a ligand-activated transcriptional factor, which regulates the expression of various genes, including enzymes responsible for xenobiotic metabolism [7].

AhR-mediates the toxicity of uncountable xenobiotics, and their triggered toxicity is accompanied by an overexpression and overactivation of AhR in cells. Thus, it increases the pathophysiological functions of AhR and could develop cancer in different organs such as the breast and liver. In addition, it can also lead to cardiovascular diseases, among other diseases [8, 9]. Thus, targeting AhR with a small molecule agonist/antagonist could efficiently inhibit several of the important hallmarks of various cancers [10].

Computational modeling and computer simulations continue to be an important tool for studying various biological mechanisms and for analyzing the interactions between biomolecular entities (*e.g.* proteins, DNA, and drugs). These methods use complex physiochemical and mathematical algorithms to predict the interactions between ligands and proteins at the atomistic level [11]. For instance, in the case of AhR, several computational studies have been reported to screen the chemical space for potential AhR modulators and to investigate how these ligands interact with the individual residues within AhR [12, 13]. This chapter will focus on summarizing the findings and computational approaches described in these studies. The chapter first discusses current knowledge related to AhR functions and describes all reported AhR crystal structures. It will then provide an overview on the different computational studies reported in the literature, which focused on investigating AhR dynamics and on identifying novel AhR modulators. We hope the information provided in this chapter can advance the development of AhR ligands and contribute to progress in this important research area.

2. AhR structure and functions

2.1 AhR domain structure

AhR is a member of the basic helix–loop–helix (bHLH)-PER- ARNT-SIM (PAS) family of transcription factors. The "PAS" term is an abbreviation for three proteins, namely, the Drosophila circadian rhythm protein period (Per), the mammalian AhR nuclear translocator (ARNT), and Drosophila neurogenic protein single-minded (Sim) [7, 14, 15]. Human AhR is a 848 amino acid with a molecular weight of ~96 kDa [16]. It includes two PAS domains, namely PAS A and PAS B, and interacts with the Aryl hydrocarbon nuclear tranlocator (ARNT) protein. Moreover, the PAS B domain involves two interactions sites: a ligand-binding site in which a bound ligand can modulate the AhR activity; and a direct binding interface for the HSP 90-chaperone protein. Additionally, AhR includes a basic helix loop helix motif located near its N-terminal domain, which is responsible for DNA binding as well as contributing to other protein–protein interactions. Finally, the transactivation (*i.e.*, glutamine-rich region) domain is located close to the C-terminal of AhR and binds to a co-activator [7] as shown in **Figure 1**.

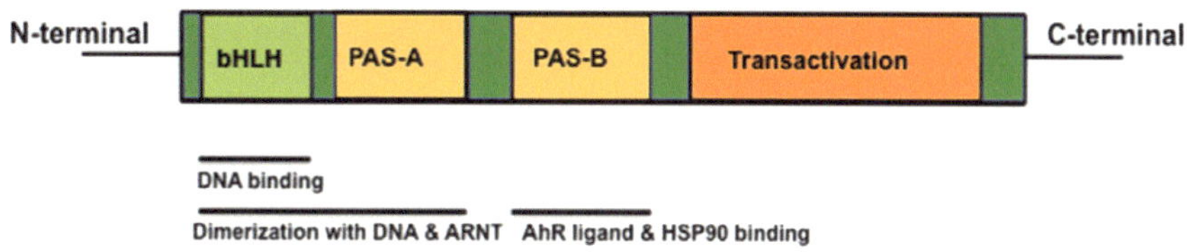

Figure 1.
AhR domain structure and sub-domains' functions.

2.2 The AhR ligands and their modes of action

The AhR PAS B domain can interact with both exogenous and endogenous chemicals from various origins. These interactions can induce different effects on AhR activity, leading to a wide range of physiological and toxicological downstream consequences. For example, several studies showed that environmental pollutants have been associated with developing cardiovascular diseases, cancer, and other diseases through AhR modulation [7, 17, 18]. Exogenous AhR ligands include various aromatic hydrocarbon molecules such as dioxins. One can be exposed to such ligands through contaminated food or environmental pollutants. Following exposure, their interaction with AhR can lead to several toxic effects, including organ dysfunctions, immunotoxicity, and carcinogenicity. On the other hand, endogenous AhR ligands are usually metabolic derivatives derived from cellular processes such as 6-Formylindolo (3,2- b) carbazole (FICZ). The interaction of these ligands with AhR is part of a normal functional response through AhR modulation [7, 19, 20].

2.3 AhR physiological and pathophysiological roles

AhR is an essential protein that contributes to countless biological pathways to establish its physiological role in developing the immune system and regulating xenobiotic enzymes [7, 15, 21]. AhR knockout mice models showed abnormal female reproductive functions and impairment in managing blood pressure [7]. The overactivation and constitutive activation of AhR have been associated with the initiation, promotion, progression, and invasion of cancer cells. For example, activating AhR by exogenous AhR ligands can have several effects, which includes inducing cell proliferation in the G1-S phase, silencing tumor suppressor genes, and activating proto-oncogenes in cancer cell lines.

Earlier findings showed that the exogenous AhR ligand, 2,3,7,8-tetrachlorodibenzo-p-dioxin TCDD promoted the degradation of cell–cell adhesion and expansion of cancer cells' motility by separating the Src kinase from the AhR protein complex. Furthermore, the activation of AhR via environmental pollutants can lead to a significant induction of xenobiotic-metabolizing enzymes, including CYP1A, which produces reactive intermediate metabolites and reactive oxygen species to promote tumor growth [14, 22]. In a nutshell, AhR resembles a machinery of genes, which controls xenobiotic-metabolizing enzymes in phases I and II, as shown in **Table 1**. Also, known AhR agonists such as TCDD and β -naphthoflavone have been shown to induce cellular hypertrophic actions on H9c2 cardiomyoblast cells. This was correlated with an increase in the levels of numerous cytochrome P450 genes, which could overcome by using an AhR antagonist [31].

On the positive side, experiments on a mouse model of induced colitis showed that the endogenous AhR agonist (FICZ), which has a strong binding affinity towards AhR, could block IL-6 and claudin-2 expression, and prevent any induced disorders in the intestinal barrier function through AhR activation [32].

Metabolism phase	Gene	Reference
Phase I	CYP1A1	[23]
Phase I	CYP1A2	[24]
Phase I	CYP1B1	[25]
Phase I	CYP2S1	[26]
Phase II	NQO1 NAD(P)H: Quinine oxidoreductase 1	[27]
Phase II	GSTA1 Glutathione transferase A1/2	[28]
Phase II	UGT1A6 Uridine diphosphate glucuronosyltransferase 1A6	[29]
Phase II	ALDH3A1 Aldehyde dehydrogenase 3A1	[30]

Table 1.
Xenobiotic metabolizing enzymes genes regulate via AhR pathway.

Further protein knockout studies showed that AhR ligands play a fundamental role in autoimmune diseases through regulating Tregs and TH17 cell differentiation in the immune system. For example, FICZ inhibited Treg and TH17 cell development, accelerating experimental autoimmune encephalomyelitis in mice models [21, 33].

2.4 AhR signaling pathways

AhR is generally expressed in its inactive form in the cytoplasm as part of a protein complex encompassing a dimer heat shock protein, co-chaperone p23, an AhR-interacting protein, called AIP, and the protein kinase SRC (see **Figure 2**). The PAS

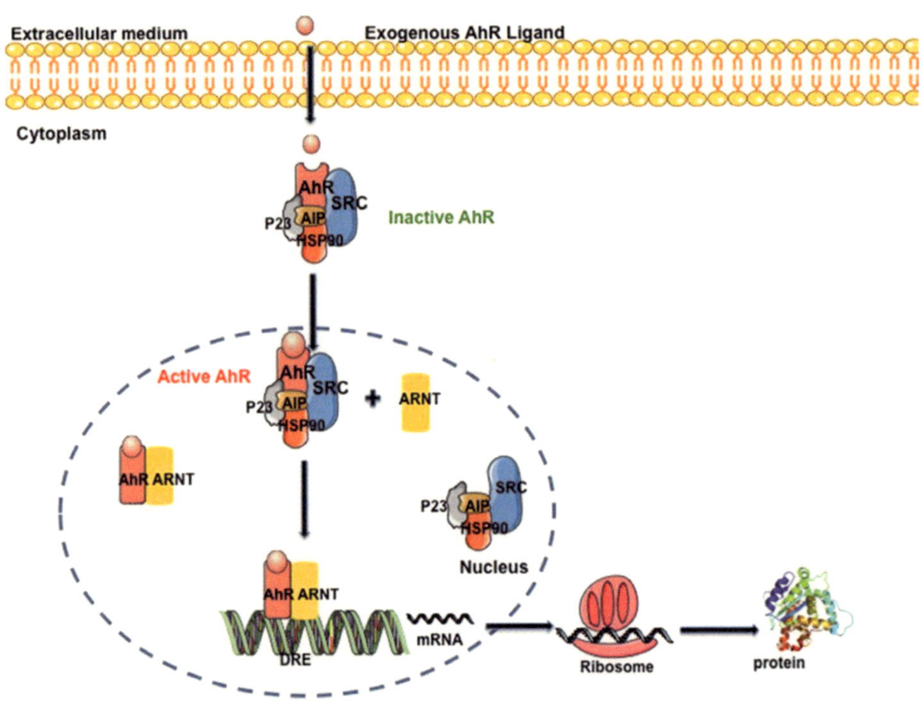

Figure 2.
Canonical pathway of aryl hydrocarbon receptor.

B domain within AhR binds to one monomer of the HSP90 dimer and the second HSP90 monomer interacts with the AhR basic helix–loop–helix domain (bHLH) as well as with the PAS A domain [34]. As shown in **Figure 2**, the bHLH domain within AhR is also crucial for DNA binding in a process initiated by the binding of an AhR ligand within the PAS B domain and its interaction with the co-chaperone P23. Binding to P23 stabilizes AhR in the cytoplasm, protecting it from proteasomal degrading, and also maintains the PAS B domain of AhR in a unique conformation, suitable for strong ligand binding [35, 36].

Once an AhR ligand binds to the PAS B domain, it forms an AhR-ligand complex, including p23, SRC, and AIP (see **Figure 2**). This complex is transformed into an active state and then translocated inside the nucleus. Then in the nucleus, all complex components dissociate from the AhR-ligand complex, excluding an agonist and AhR protein. Subsequently, AhR forms an active heterodimer with ARNT and creates an AhR–ARNT complex. This complex is then recruited to the DNA via the Dioxin response element (DRE), exhibiting a common DNA compromise motif (5′-TNGCGTG-3). This canonical AhR pathway increases the expression of various genes, including the principal ones in xenobiotic metabolism, AhR repressor (AHRR), and other genes [36].

3. AhR three-dimensional structures

Resolving the full-length three-dimensional structure of AhR has been a challenging exercise for the last two decades. Unfortunately, despite the many efforts towards this goal, there is no complete structure for the whole AhR protein. However, as discussed below, there are a few structures, which describe the number AhR domains. Although these structures do not reveal the exact overall AhR architecture, they can still provide useful information on the function of these separate domains. Giving computational modeling a favorable vantage point to construct reliable hypotheses for the full-length AhR organization for rational drug development and drug screening campaigns.

The first AHR 3D structure was reported in 2013 for the mouse PAS A domain (residues 110 to 267) at a resolution of 2.55 Å (PDB ID: 4M4X) (see **Figure 3**). This X-ray diffraction-based PAS A homodimer structure was obtained from recombinant *E. coli* expression. It contained a five β-sheet and elements order B-A-I-H-G, with four α-helices (Cα, Dα, Eα, and Fα) adjoining one side of the β-sheet. The interactions between the two PAS A monomers involved two distinctive areas within the A′ α-helices, revealing a strong interaction between Phe115, Leu116, and Ala119 from the A′ α-helix in one monomer with Val124, Phe260, and Ile262 from the β-sheet in the other monomer as shown in **Figure 3**. The protein structure revealed an undruggable pocket due to hydrophobic residues, and other residues such as Gln112 and Ile262 are essential in the interface for AHR dimerization, either homodimer or heterodimer with ARNT [37, 38].

Two more additional AhR structures were revealed in 2017 (see **Figure 4**). The two structures comprise multiple AhR domains and show a clear interaction between AhR and its dimerization partner, ARNT, as well as its interaction with two DNA strands. The two structures (PDB IDs: 5V0L and 5NJ8) [39, 40] were resolved at a resolution of 4.0 and 3.35 Å, respectively and revealed the complex formation among the bHLH and PAS A domains from human AhR and their interactions with ARNT and DNA. However, due to the observed high flexibility of the AhR PAS B domain and the transactive domain (C- terminal), none of these two subdomains were included in this architecture. However, both structures clearly explain the protein–protein interactions (PPI) and show clear interface regions for these

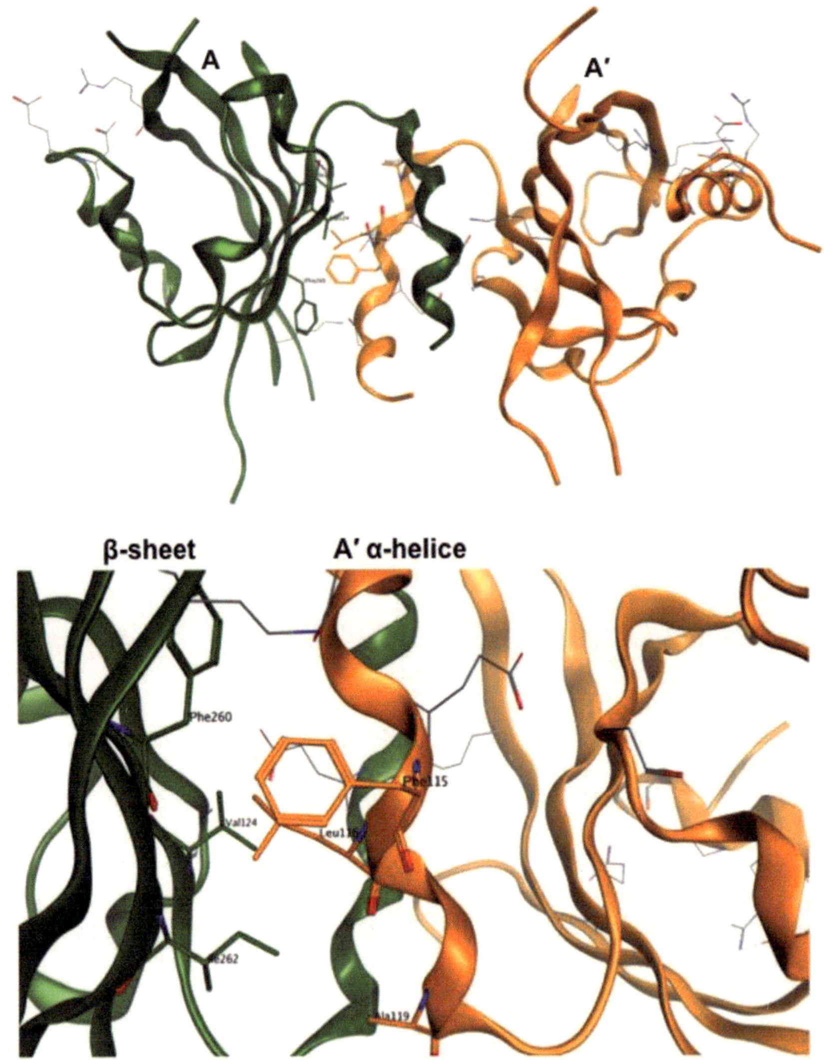

Figure 3.
The upper figure represents crystal structure of homodimer mouse AhR-PAS a obtained from protein databank [37], and the lower figure shows the interactions between the two monomers.

interactions between the individual domains within AhR as well as their interactions with ARNET and DNA.

As shown in **Figure 4**, the first PPI interface is between the AhR-ARNT heterodimer with the two DNA strands. This interaction is mediated by DRE Ser36, His39, and Arg40 from the AhR bHLH domain and His79, Asp83, Arg86, and Arg87 from ARNT, as well as thymine and guanine from the DNA. The second PPI interface is between AhR and ARNT through different regions within the two proteins. These regions involve many hydrophobic interactions from both proteins and comprise residues Leu47, Leu50, Leu53, Val74, and Leu70 from the AhR bHLH domain and residues Ile109, Leu112, Val136, and Met139 in ARNT. The third PPI interface involves interactions between residues from the PAS A domain in both AhR and ARNT, mediated by residues Phe117, Leu118, Ala121, Leu122, Tyr137, Val126, Phe266, and Ile268 from AhR. The fourth, and final PPI interface encompasses the interdomain interactions between the AhR bHLH

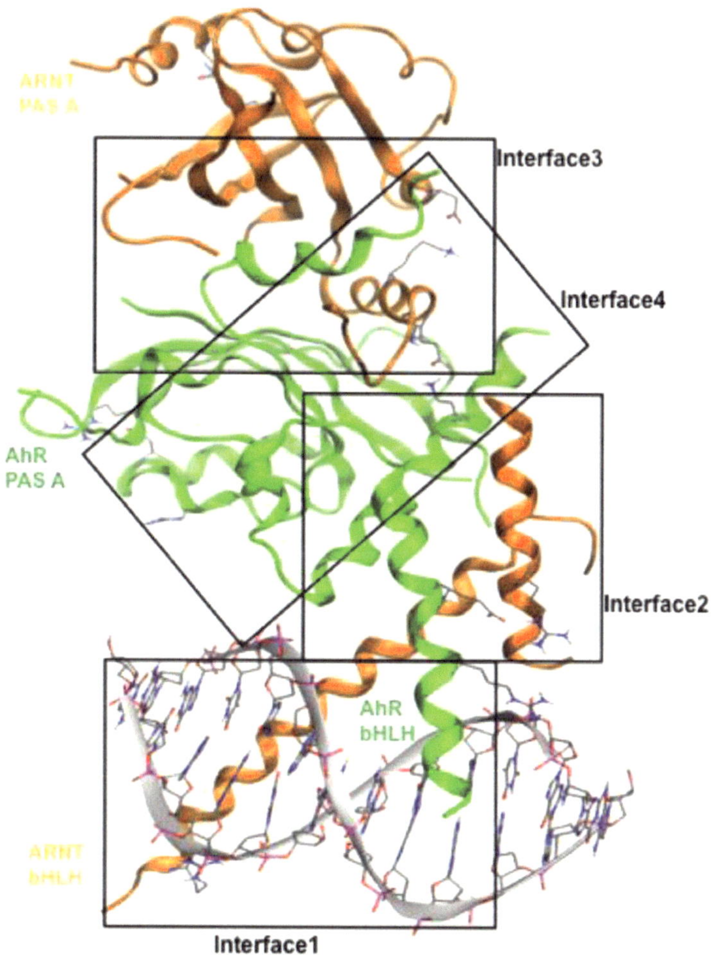

Figure 4.
Crystal structure of human aryl hydrocarbon receptor in heterodimer with aryl hydrocarbon nuclear translocator and recruit on DNA in dioxin element response [39].

and AhR PAS A domains, through residues Phe136, Ser151, Ile154, and Leu246 from the PAS A domain and Phe56, Val60, Leu72, Ala79, and Phe82 from the bHLH domain.

4. Applications of computational methods in AhR modeling

The wealth of structural information described above on AhR provides an excellent opportunity to apply various computer-based simulations to study the dynamicity and structural organization of the various AhR domains. The applications of such computational tools not only can yield much needed insights on how these domains interact together within the AhR machinery, but can also offer detailed answers on their interactions with other AhR partners (*e.g.* ARNT, DNA, and chaperone proteins). It can also explain how a small molecule ligand can bind to AhR and how this can affect AhR functions, conformational dynamics or its interaction with other entities. Computational tools can also suggest novel-binding sites either within the AhR structure, or at the interfaces described above to either stabilize these interaction (*i.e.* agonism) or block these interactions (*i.e.* antagonism). Most importantly, computational methods including virtual screening can be used as a high throughput-screening tool to identify compounds that can bind to these sites to modulate the AhR activity.

4.1 Modeling the PAS B domain

Most of the *in silico* AhR screening campaigns till now focused on studying the PAS B domain. The PAS B domain is also known as the ligand-binding domain (LBD), where the ligands (agonists/antagonists) have been shown to bind [41]. Given that the available AhR structures (described above) lack this domain, computational methods played a key role in studying the interactions of ligands with this important region. Towards this goal, homology modeling was used to build 3-dimensional structures for this domain to allow the study of ligand binding to AhR. A homology model approach usually starts with identifying a similar template to the target domain (*i.e.*, the PAS B domain in this case). Once a template is identified, one uses various computational methods (*e.g.* sequence alignment, threading, and loop modeling) to construct the 3-dimensional structure of the target protein [42].

In many AhR studies, the human hypoxia inducible factors (HIF-2α) crystal structures served as templates for AhR-PAS B domain because it has the highest sequence similarity towards the AhR-PAS B domain. **Table 2** provides a list of the reported *in silico* studies that were conducted over the last few years by adopting various crystal structures of HIF-2α as starting points to construct PAS B models. These studies were focused on understanding the roles played by the different PAS B residues in interacting with known AhR modulators and to screen for novel AhR ligands. Docking findings from these studies indicated that the binding cavity within the AhR-LBD can accommodate ligands with structural maximal dimensions of 14 A° X 12 A° X 5A°, and showed that their binding within AhR relies mainly on electronic properties [17]. Given this information, various computational methods including molecular modeling, molecular docking followed by MD simulations, and binding free energy calculations were used to provide insights about ligand interactions within the PAS B pockets [49].

For example, Bisson and his group established an agonist-optimized model of the human AhR-PAS B domain, followed by docking around five thousand chemical structures, including AhR agonists and antagonists, within the PAS B domain.

PDB ID	Structure method	Year of study	Reference
3H82	X-ray diffraction	2014	[41]
4GHI	X-ray diffraction	2014	[43]
3H3W	Electron microscopy	2016	[44]
3F1O, 3H7W, 3H82	X-ray diffraction	2018, 2018	[45, 46]
4XT2	X-ray diffraction	2019	[47]
3F1N, 3F1O, 3F1P, 3H7W, 3H82, 4GHI, 4GS9, 4XT2, 4ZP4, 4ZQD	X-ray diffraction	2019	[12]
3H82, 3H7W, 4ZQD	X-ray diffraction	2020	[48]

Table 2.
Report studies that used different crystal structures of human hypoxia inducible factors (HIF-2α).

Docking results were then filtered and the top five systems were subjected to long MD simulations (~ 60 ns) to study the conformational and dynamical changes in these generated complexes. Findings from Bisson's work revealed the importance of residues 307–329 in the PAS B domain, which were shown to be very flexible, acting as an access gate to the ligand-binding pocket. These residues can also adopt different conformations upon AhR ligands' binding and play a primary function in controlling the structural changes and accessibility of the ligands to the AhR ligand binding pocket [41].

4.2 Interaction of the PAS B domain with different ligands

With the 3-dimensional structure of the PAS B domain in hand, many groups focused on studying its binding to different ligands (*e.g.*, TCDD) (shown in **Figure 5**) [50] and investigated this binding reaction for different species. For example, TCDD studies on mouse AhR revealed a number of conserved residues that regulate the access of TCDD to the binding pocket [51–53]. These residues include Thr283, His285, Phe289, Tyr316, Ile319, Cys327, Met334, Phe345, Ala375, and Gln377 and have been also shown to control the internal size of the binding cavity [54–56]. Similarly, aromatic side chains of Phe 289, Phe 345, and Tyr 316 were shown to be important in stabilizing TCDD in its best mode of binding via non-covalent interaction [54].

Mutations at outer residues (e.g., Arg282, Thr311, Glu339, and Lys350) into alanine did not impact TCDD binding to AhR [57]. In the human AHR-LBD a mutation at Ala375 to Val and Leu decreases the binding affinity of TCDD and makes indirubin a less potent endogenous AhR ligand [45, 58]. Additional site-directed mutagenesis within AhR-LBD residues has been used to identify key residues promoting for ligand selectivity in AhR. These developed models provided a clear basis towards understanding the mechanism of ligand-dependent activation of AHR via its PAS B domain. In particular, the above mentioned molecular docking

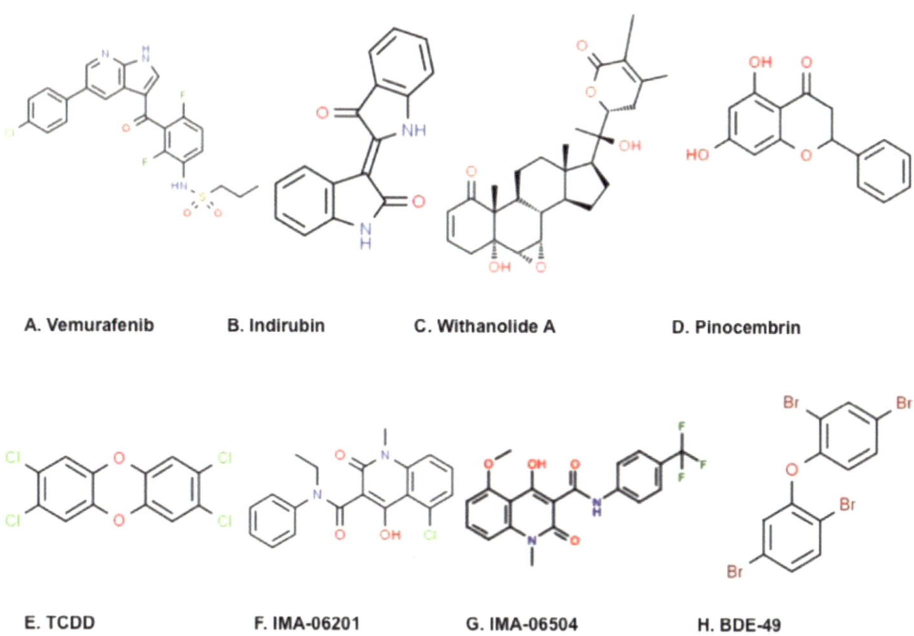

Figure 5.
Chemical structures of AhR ligands in this study obtained from pubchem database.

and mutagenesis analyses helped in identifying and confirming the binding pocket of TCDD and other AhR modulators [52, 57, 59, 60].

Examples of these models include those developed by Kim and her team, who constructed 3D models from several avian species including, chicken, albatross, and cormorant, and studied the sensitivity of dioxin derivatives against multiple AhR isoforms. All models were subjected to docking simulations with TCDD followed by MD simulations. Kim's results used the mean square displacement (MSD) of the MD trajectories as a stability indicator for the bound ligands. These findings revealed Ile324 and Ser380 from chicken AhR1 exhibited the least MSD values compared to all AhR-LBD residues in other avian species. The size of binding pocket was also shown to be variable among the different species. Moreover, stabilization of TCDD in the binding pocket of chicken AhR relied on the features of Ile324 and Ser380, which explained why chicken AhR is more sensitive to TCDD binding compared to other AhR isoforms [54, 61–63].

Further mutational and functional analysis studies were expanded to include additional AhR modulators other than TCCD. For example, the work of Faber and her team studied induribin binding to AhR in both mouse and human. This study revealed that a mutation in His326Tyr and Ala349Thr in mouse AhR, and Tyr332 and Thr355 in human AhR can increase the potency of indole compounds, particularly, indirubin. Also, although indirubin and vemurafenib can fit within the same binding pocket in AhR, the two compounds showed two different modes of binding [45, 47]. For example, flutamide efficiently binds to residues inside the AHR-LBD with a high affinity in both mouse and human AHR to activate the AhR pathway [64]. It is important to note that, the biological response of AhR is dependant on the type of the bound ligand and has been shown to change based on the interaction of a given ligand with the residues forming the LBD in the PAS B domain [48, 65].

4.3 Virtual screening and machine learning models applied to AhR

Over the last few decades, virtual screening has been used as a major tool to in hit identification campaigns against numerous biological targets [66]. In this regard, AhR is no exception and various *in silico* screening methods have been employed to identify new AhR modulators based on the developed 3D models for the PAS B domain [13]. These methods can be classified into two major groups; ligand-based methods (*e.g.,* quantitative structure–activity relationship (QSAR)) and structure-based methods (*e.g.,* docking and MD simulations). Ligand-based methods (LB) depend on the knowledge of known active/inactive molecules against a given target or disease to suggest new active chemical entities. Ligand-based methods are typically used when no information about the 3D structure of the target is available. They include QSAR, pharmacophore modeling and machine learning algorithms methods. QSAR models, for example, correlates the structural, physicochemical features, and biological mode of action of known compounds to build a mathematical model, which can be used to suggest new modifications to these structures for better activity or improved biophysical/biochemical properties [67–69].

Pharmacophore modeling maps the ligand-target interactions into a set of steric and electronic features structured in a specific 3D arrangement [70]. These pharmacophore models can be then used to screen millions of available chemical structural libraries for compounds that satisfy these pharmacophore features, which can be used for scaffold hopping and fragment-based drug design. On the other hand, structure–based methods require the knowledge of target protein crystal structure, or its 3D developed homology models. Ligands from a given database can be fitted into the active site of the target protein and can be ranked based on the predicted binding affinities. In this context, molecular docking and molecular dynamics simulations are among the many valuable tools that can be used to predict the most probable mode of binding of a given ligand within the target. Furthermore, structure-based pharmacophore models can provide more detailed insights on the interaction of ligand with the binding site [69, 71, 72].

As discussed below, several AhR screening studies combined both methods to enhance the search for possible AhR candidates [67, 73]. The plethora of accumulated physicochemical, chemical and structural data on AhR modulators augmented this hit identification search with great tools to build reliable machine learning models, which require large datasets of chemical structures along with their interaction kinetics with AhR [74].

An example of AhR *in silico* screening studies is the one implemented by Xiao et al., who constructed 3D structures of the PAS B using the HIF-2α as a template. Xiao used his model to study the effects of ~185 polybrominated diphenyl ethers (PBDEs), classified as organic pollutants, on AhR activation. This study combined molecular docking simulations, two-dimensional quantitative structure–activity relationship (2D-QSAR) models, and three-dimensional QSAR (3D-QSAR) models to analyze the local ligands' interactions against a diverse set of PAS B configurations. Their result showed that bromide replacements in at the ortho- or meta-positions of PBDEs (BDE-49) as shown in the **Figure 5** exhibited the largest effect on PBDEs' binding, mainly interacting with residues Met342, Thr290, Met334, and Phe289 in the binding site of the AHR-PAS B model in mouse and zebrafish [75, 76].

In a similar approach, Rath and his team built two human PAS B domain; a wild type and mutant (Val381 Ala, Val381Asn) models. Around 60 natural compounds from *Withania somnifera* were then docked within these models. Docking rustles were then refined using MD simulations for 50 ns. Findings from Rath's study showed that withaferin A, withanolide A, withanolide B, withanolide D and withanone were effective as AhR ligands in all three models. In the meantime, withanolide A was more stable in the binding site and interacted with various residues in each model even after 50 ns of the MD simulations. Withanolide A was further validated experimentally in an *in vivo* zebrafish model to significantly reduce CYP1A1 expression. This was done in the presence of a strong AhR activator, namely benzo[a]pyrene in adult zebrafish brain when administrated together. Thus, withanolide A (see **Figure 5** and **Table 3**) neutralized the benzo[a]pyrene toxicity in zebrafish brain [77].

Compound name	Induction of AhR transcription	Binding free energy (kcal/mol)	Reference
Withanolide A	+	−7.5	[77]
Pinocembrin (5,7-Dihydroxyflavanone, R-form)	+	−2.9	[60]
5-hydroxy-7-methoxyflavone	+	−4.3	[60]
IMA-06201 (N-ethyl-*N*-phenyl-5-chloro-1,2-dihydro-4-hydroxy-1-methyl-2-oxo-quinoline-3-carboxamide)	+	Not report	[46]
IMA-06504 (N-(4-trifluoromethylphenyl)-1,2-dihydro-4-hydroxy-5-methoxy-1-methyl-2-oxo-quinoline-3-carboxamide)	+	Not report	[46]

Table 3.
Activation of AhR transcription by chemical compounds that identified by in silico screening of different chemical libraries.

In another screening study, Mahiout, et al. identified IMA-06201 and IMA-06504 as two novel AhR agonists, with similar modes of binding to that of TCDD. Both compounds showed great stability in the central area of the AhR ligand-binding pocket. Furthermore, these AhR agonists were shown to be more efficient and more potent as selective AhR modulators than TCDD. To confirm that, Mahiout used CYP1A1 enzyme activity as a biomarker for AhR activation and compared the efficacy and potency of IMA-06201 and IMA-06504 (see **Figure 5** and **Table 3**) to that of TCDD in the presence and absence of the AhR antagonist, CH-223191, at different concentrations in rat hepatoma cell lines. Their results showed that the new compounds, IMA-06201 and IMA-06504, were able to induce CYP1A1 activity in a similar efficacy to that of TCDD, where CH-223191 was shown to block their CYP1A1 induction. Also, in an Ames test to assess the genotoxicity of the new identified compounds, IMA-06201 and IMA-06504 did not show mutagenic effects at low concentrations [46].

Machine-learning algorithms combined with QSAR have been recently used to screen for new AhR ligands. For instance, Matsuzaka used deep learning (DL) to construct machine-learning models to predict AhR activators. These models showed advantages on enhanced input data based on the 3D chemical structures of the compounds into these models, and their performance was better than traditional machine learning models [78]. To enhance the screening process of AhR ligands, Zhu established a virtual screening protocol from combining ligand-based and structure-based screening with supervised machine learning to screen around eight thousand from the pesticide databases to identify an agonistic effect on AHR activity. Zhu's results revealed sixteen compounds as AhR activators and these findings were validated in a zebrafish *in vivo* model to assess their AhR activation and exhibited induction in CYP 1a1 levels [79].

Towards improving the prediction accuracy of his model, Yang, et al. used machine learning algorithms to construct two-dimensional quantitative structure–activity relationship (2D-QSAR) models from multiple linear regression (MLR) and artificial neural network (ANN) algorithms. He used the pEC50 values of 60 dioxins derivatives as AhR activators to build. These models predicted the toxicity of 162 new dioxin derivatives, showing a good correlation between compounds' chemical structures and their IC50 and EC50 values.

Recently, Goya-Jorge employed various machine learning algorithms to build a set of QSAR models. These models adopted the adoboost (AdB), random forest (RF), gradient boosting (GB), support vector machine (SVM), and multilayer perceptron (MLP) as classifiers to examine around 1900 compounds from synthetic and natural sources on their AhR agonism. Around 40 compounds baring the benzothiazole scaffold were classified as AhR agonists. In vitro validation of these hits showed that indole derivatives can serve as AhR ligands, including the endogenous substances [80, 81]. **Table 3** reports some of the top hits emerging from different *in silico* studies.

5. Current challenges in modeling AhR

Identifying novel AhR modulators using in silico approaches require establishing more comprehensive computational models of this target. These models should describe the detailed organization of the different AhR domains as well is its interaction with other protein/DNA partners. While the available crystal structures provide a glimpse of these missing pieces of information, there are still more to be done in this regard. For example, all currently available AhR crystal structures deposited in the protein data bank are lacking two important AhR domains, namely the PAS B domain and the transactivation domain [39]. The transactivation domain is essential in AhR intercellular trafficking.

On the other hand, the PAS B domain interacts with an AhR ligand, which can modulate the AhR activity. While homology modeling has helped constructing acceptable models for this domain, the similarity of the templates used to build the PAS B domain is very low, leaving a lot of doubt about their accuracy. A crystal structure of the PAS B domain would be a great leap forward towards understanding the mode of action of AhR modulators and towards identifying better agonists/antagonists for this important target. Furthermore, there is a gap of knowledge on how AhR interact with other protein partners in the inactive state, including co-chaperone, AIP, and the protein kinase SRC. This builds an additional challenge to identify druggable pockets at their protein–protein interfaces [7, 82]. With the apparent advances in obtaining 3D experimental structures of protein (e.g. Cryo-electron microscopy (cryo-EM)) one expects several of these structural challenges can be solved in the near future, opening new gates for the computational science to identify new AhR modulators and to help understand its functional, structural and biological characterizes more clearly.

6. Executive summary

The AhR is a ligand-activated transcriptional factor. It regulates various genes' expression and plays a pathophysiological function in numerous diseases. Crystallography has been employed to resolve three crystal structures containing bHLH and PAS A domains from human and mouse origin and to identify four protein–protein interfaces. However, all these structures lacked the PAS B domain, which plays a fundamental role in ligands' binding domain to AhR. Computational and mutational studies revealed important residues that constitute the binding pockets within the PAS B domain. Towards identifying novel AhR modulators, several virtual screening and machine learning algorithms were constructed based on the available structural and pharmacological properties of known AhR ligands. Computational methods are extremely fast and intensely reduce the cost and time in screening millions of compounds to find compounds that could interact with the AhR. Recent studies employing these methods against AhR have been reviewed and discussed in this chapter. We hope the literature presented here can help advance the development of novel, selective and potent AhR modulators.

Author details

Farag E.S. Mosa, Ayman O.S. El-Kadi* and Khaled Barakat*
Faculty of Pharmacy and Pharmaceutical Sciences, University of Alberta, Edmonton, AB, Canada

*Address all correspondence to: kbarakat@ualberta.ca and aelkadi@ualberta.ca

References

[1] A.H. Conney, J.J. Burns, Stimulatory effect of foreign compounds on ascorbic acid biosynthesis and on drug-metabolizing enzymes, Nature. 184 (1959) 363-364. doi:10.1038/184363a0.

[2] A. Poland, E. Glover, A.K.-J. of B. Chemistry, undefined 1976, Stereospecific, high affinity binding of 2, 3, 7, 8-tetrachlorodibenzo-p-dioxin by hepatic cytosol. Evidence that the binding species is receptor for induction of Elsevier. (n.d.). https://www.sciencedirect.com/science/article/pii/S0021925817332052 (accessed January 24, 2021).

[3] Y.Z. Jiang, K. Wang, R. Fang, J. Zheng, Expression of aryl hydrocarbon receptor in human placentas and fetal tissues, J. Histochem. Cytochem. 58 (2010) 679-685. doi:10.1369/jhc.2010.955955.

[4] K.M. Burbach, A. Poland, C.A. Bradfield, Cloning of the Ah-receptor cDNA reveals a distinctive ligand-activated transcription factor., Proc. Natl. Acad. Sci. U. S. A. 89 (1992) 8185-8189. doi:10.1073/pnas.89.17.8185.

[5] P. Fernandez-Salguero, T. Pineau, D.M. Hilbert, T. McPhail, S.S.T. Lee, S. Kimura, D.W. Nebert, S. Rudikoff, J.M. Ward, F.J. Gonzalez, Immune system impairment and hepatic fibrosis in mice lacking the dioxin-binding Ah receptor, Science (80-.). 268 (1995) 722-726. doi:10.1126/science.7732381.

[6] K.W. Bock, Human and rodent aryl hydrocarbon receptor (AHR): From mediator of dioxin toxicity to physiologic AHR functions and therapeutic options, Biol. Chem. 398 (2017) 455-464. doi:10.1515/hsz-2016-0303.

[7] L. Larigot, L. Juricek, J. Dairou, X. Coumoul, AhR signaling pathways and regulatory functions, Biochim. Open. 7 (2018) 1-9. doi:10.1016/j.biopen.2018.05.001.

[8] I.A. Murray, A.D. Patterson, G.H. Perdew, Aryl hydrocarbon receptor ligands in cancer: Friend and foe, Nat. Rev. Cancer. 14 (2014) 801-814. doi:10.1038/nrc3846.

[9] C. Esser, A. Rannug, The aryl hydrocarbon receptor in barrier organ physiology, immunology, and toxicology, Pharmacol. Rev. 67 (2015) 259-279. doi:10.1124/pr.114.009001.

[10] S.K. Kolluri, U.H. Jin, S. Safe, Role of the aryl hydrocarbon receptor in carcinogenesis and potential as an anti-cancer drug target, Arch. Toxicol. 91 (2017) 2497-2513. doi:10.1007/s00204-017-1981-2.

[11] A. Ganesan, K. Barakat, Applications of computer-aided approaches in the development of hepatitis C antiviral agents, Expert Opin. Drug Discov. 12 (2017) 407-425. doi:10.1080/17460441.2017.1291628.

[12] S. Giani Tagliabue, S.C. Faber, S. Motta, M.S. Denison, L. Bonati, Modeling the binding of diverse ligands within the Ah receptor ligand binding domain, Sci. Rep. 9 (2019) 1-14. doi:10.1038/s41598-019-47138-z.

[13] X. Lin, X. Li, X. Lin, A review on applications of computational methods in drug screening and design, Molecules. 25 (2020). doi:10.3390/molecules25061375.

[14] J.P. Whitlock, Induction of cytochrome P4501A1, Annu. Rev. Pharmacol. Toxicol. 39 (1999) 103-125. doi:10.1146/annurev.pharmtox.39.1.103.

[15] T. V. Beischlag, J.L. Morales, B.D. Hollingshead, G.H. Perdew, The aryl hydrocarbon receptor complex and the control of gene expression, Crit. Rev.

Eukaryot. Gene Expr. 18 (2008) 207-250. doi:10.1615/CritRevEukarGeneExpr.v18.i3.20.

[16] C. Rowlands, J.C. Rowlandsar, J.-A. Gustafssonbj, Aryl Hydrocarbon Receptor-Mediated Signal Transduction, Aryl Hydrocarbon Receptor-Mediated Signal Transduct ion Artic. Crit. Rev. Toxicol. 27 (1997) 109-110. doi:10.3109/10408449709021615.

[17] J. Abel, T. Haarmann-Stemmann, An introduction to the molecular basics of aryl hydrocarbon receptor biology, Biol. Chem. 391 (2010) 1235-1248. doi:10.1515/BC.2010.128.

[18] E.M. Reyes-Reyes, I.N. Ramos, M.A. Tavera-Garcia, K.S. Ramos, The aryl hydrocarbon receptor agonist benzo(a) pyrene reactivates LINE-1 in HepG2 cells through canonical TGF-β1 signaling: Implications in hepatocellular carcinogenesis, Am. J. Cancer Res. 6 (2016) 1066-1077.

[19] O. Ibraheem, T.H. Fatoki, J.M. Enibukun, B.C. Faleye, D.U. Momodu, In silico toxicological analyzes of selected toxic compounds from dumpsite or contaminated soils on human health, Nov. Biotechnol. Chim. 18 (2019) 144-153. doi:10.2478/nbec-2019-0017.

[20] M. Adam, L. Chaubah, B.W. Bontes, N.A. Mulachelah, J. Veteran, M. East, J. Indonesia, Molecular Docking of Polycyclic Aromatic Hydrocarbons as Potentially Carcinogenic Molecules Through Binding with Aryl Hydrocarbon Receptor, J. Smart Bioprospecting Technol. P-ISSN. 01 (2019) 1. https://doi.org/10.21776/ub.jsmartech.2019.001.01.

[21] F.J. Quintana, A.S. Basso, A.H. Iglesias, T. Korn, M.F. Farez, E. Bettelli, M. Caccamo, M. Oukka, H.L. Weiner, Control of Treg and TH17 cell differentiation by the aryl hydrocarbon receptor, Nature. 453 (2008) 65-71. doi:10.1038/nature06880.

[22] P. Xue, J. Fu, Y. Zhou, The aryl hydrocarbon receptor and tumor immunity, Front. Immunol. 9 (2018) 1. doi:10.3389/fimmu.2018.00286.

[23] F. Saatcioglu, D.J. Perry, D.S. Pasco, J.B. Fagan, Multiple DNA-binding factors interact with overlapping specificities at the aryl hydrocarbon response element of the cytochrome P450IA1 gene., Mol. Cell. Biol. 10 (1990) 6408-6416. doi:10.1128/mcb.10.12.6408.

[24] W. Li, P.A. Harper, B.K. Tang, A.B. Okey, Regulation of cytochrome P450 enzymes by aryl hydrocarbon receptor in human cells. CYP1A2 expression in the LS180 colon carcinoma cell line after treatment with 2,3,7,8-tetrachlorodibenzo-p-dioxin or 3-methylcholanthrene, Biochem. Pharmacol. 56 (1998) 599-612. doi:10.1016/S0006-2952(98)00208-1.

[25] L. Zhang, Ü. Savas, D.L. Alexander, C.R. Jefcoate, Characterization of the mouse Cyp1B1 gene: Identification of an enhancer region that directs aryl hydrocarbon receptor-mediated constitutive and induced expression: J. Biol. Chem. 273 (1998) 5174-5183. doi:10.1074/jbc.273.9.5174.

[26] S.P. Rivera, S.T. Saarikoski, O. Hankinson, Identification of a novel dioxin-inducible cytochrome P450, Mol. Pharmacol. 61 (2002) 255-259. doi:10.1124/mol.61.2.255.

[27] L. V. Favreau, C.B. Pickett, Transcriptional regulation of the rat NAD(P)H:Quinone reductase gene. Characterization of a DNA-protein interaction at the antioxidant responsive element and induction by 12-O-tetradecanoylphorbol 13-acetate, J. Biol. Chem. 268 (1993) 19875-19881. doi:10.1016/s0021-9258(19)36594-9.

[28] M. Rojas, I. Cascorbi, K. Alexandrov, E. Kriek, G. Auburtin, L. Mayer, A. Kopp-Schneider, I. Roots, Modulation of benzo[a]pyrene

diolepoxide-DNA adduct levels in human white blood cells by CYP1A1, GSTM1 and GSTT1 polymorphism, 2000.

[29] M.F. Yueh, Y.H. Huang, A. Hiller, S. Chen, N. Nguyen, R.H. Tukey, Involvement of the xenobiotic response element (XRE) in Ah receptor-mediated induction of human UDP-glucuronosyltransferase 1A1, J. Biol. Chem. 278 (2003) 15001-15006. doi:10.1074/jbc.M300645200.

[30] W.T. Kays, J. Piatigorsky, Aldehyde dehydrogenase class 3 expression: Identification of a cornea-preferred gene promoter in transgenic mice, Proc. Natl. Acad. Sci. U. S. A. 94 (1997) 13594-13599. doi:10.1073/pnas.94.25.13594.

[31] B.N.M. Zordoky, A.O.S. El-Kadi, 2, 3,7,8-Tetrachlorodibenzo-p-dioxin and β-naphthoflavone induce cellular hypertrophy in H9c2 cells by an aryl hydrocarbon receptor-dependant mechanism, Toxicol. Vitr. 24 (2010) 863-871. doi:10.1016/j.tiv.2009.12.002.

[32] Y. Ma, Q. Wang, K. Yu, X. Fan, W. Xiao, Y. Cai, P. Xu, M. Yu, H. Yang, 6-Formylindolo(3,2-b)carbazole induced aryl hydrocarbon receptor activation prevents intestinal barrier dysfunction through regulation of claudin-2 expression, Chem. Biol. Interact. 288 (2018) 83-90. https://doi.org/10.1016/j.cbi.2018.04.020.

[33] B. Tong, X. Yuan, Y. Dou, X. Wu, G. Chou, Z. Wang, Y. Xia, Y. Dai, Norisoboldine, an isoquinoline alkaloid, acts as an aryl hydrocarbon receptor ligand to induce intestinal Treg cells and thereby attenuate arthritis, Int. J. Biochem. Cell Biol. 75 (2016) 63-73. doi:10.1016/j.biocel.2016.03.014.

[34] B.N. Fukunaga, M.R. Probst, S. Reisz-Porszasz, O. Hankinson, Identification of functional domains of the aryl hydrocarbon receptor, J. Biol. Chem. 270 (1995) 29270-29278. doi:10.1074/jbc.270.49.29270.

[35] I. Pongratz, G.G.F. Mason, L. Poellinger, Dual roles of the 90-kDa heat shock protein hsp90 in modulating functional activities of the dioxin receptor. Evidence that the dioxin receptor functionally belongs to a subclass of nuclear receptors which require hsp90 both for ligand binding activity and repression of intrinsic DNA binding activity, J. Biol. Chem. 267 (1992) 13728-13734. doi:10.1016/s0021-9258(18)42274-0.

[36] V. Rothhammer, F.J. Quintana, The aryl hydrocarbon receptor: an environmental sensor integrating immune responses in health and disease, Nat. Rev. Immunol. 19 (2019) 184-197. doi:10.1038/s41577-019-0125-8.

[37] D. Wu, N. Potluri, Y. Kim, F. Rastinejad, Structure and Dimerization Properties of the Aryl Hydrocarbon Receptor PAS-A Domain, Mol. Cell. Biol. 33 (2013) 4346-4356. doi:10.1128/mcb.00698-13.

[38] J. V. De Souza, S. Reznikov, R. Zhu, A.K. Bronowska, Druggability assessment of mammalian Per-Arnt-Sim [PAS] domains using computational approaches, Medchemcomm. 10 (2019) 1126-1137. doi:10.1039/c9md00148d.

[39] K.W. Schulte, E. Green, A. Wilz, M. Platten, O. Daumke, Structural Basis for Aryl Hydrocarbon Receptor-Mediated Gene Activation, Structure. 25 (2017) 1025-1033.e3. doi:10.1016/j.str.2017.05.008.

[40] S.H. Seok, W. Lee, L. Jiang, K. Molugu, A. Zheng, Y. Li, S. Park, C.A. Bradfield, Y. Xing, Structural hierarchy controlling dimerization and target DNA recognition in the AHR transcriptional complex, Proc. Natl. Acad. Sci. U. S. A. 114 (2017) 5431-5436. doi:10.1073/pnas.1617035114.

[41] A. Perkins, J. Phillips, N. Kerkvliet, R. Tanguay, G. Perdew, S. Kolluri, W. Bisson, A Structural Switch between Agonist and Antagonist Bound Conformations for a Ligand-Optimized Model of the Human Aryl Hydrocarbon Receptor Ligand Binding Domain, Biology (Basel). 3 (2014) 645-669. doi:10.3390/biology3040645.

[42] H. Jalily Hasani, K. Hassan Barakat, H. Jalily Hasani, K. Barakat, Homology Modeling: an Overview of Fundamentals and Tools Article in International Review on Modelling and Simulations · Computational drug design and molecular dynamics View project Interferon lambda signaling in the context of influenza vaccination View project Homology Modeling: an Overview of Fundamentals and Tools Int. Rev. Model. Simulations. 10 (2017). https://doi.org/10.15866/iremos.v10i2.11412.

[43] A.J. Parks, M.P. Pollastri, M.E. Hahn, E.A. Stanford, O. Novikov, D.G. Franks, S.E. Haigh, S. Narasimhan, T.D. Ashton, T.G. Hopper, D. Kozakov, D. Beglov, S. Vajda, J.J. Schlezinger, D.H. Sherr, In silico identification of an aryl hydrocarbon receptor antagonist with biological activity in vitro and in vivo, Mol. Pharmacol. 86 (2014) 593-608. doi:10.1124/mol.114.093369.

[44] I.S. Kim, J.H. Hwang, M. Hirano, H. Iwata, E.Y. Kim, In vitro and in silico evaluation of transactivation potencies of avian AHR1 and AHR2 by endogenous ligands: Implications for the physiological role of avian AHR2, Comp. Biochem. Physiol. Part - C Toxicol. Pharmacol. 187 (2016) 1-9. doi:10.1016/j.cbpc.2016.03.011.

[45] S. Faber, A. Soshilov, S. Giani Tagliabue, L. Bonati, M. Denison, Comparative In Vitro and In Silico Analysis of the Selectivity of Indirubin as a Human Ah Receptor Agonist, Int. J. Mol. Sci. 19 (2018) 2692. doi:10.3390/ijms19092692.

[46] S. Mahiout, S.G. Tagliabue, A. Nasri, I.M. Omoruyi, L. Pettersson, L. Bonati, R. Pohjanvirta, In vitro toxicity and in silico docking analysis of two novel selective AH-receptor modulators, Toxicol. Vitr. 52 (2018) 178-188. doi:10.1016/j.tiv.2018.06.010.

[47] H.C. Hawerkamp, A. Kislat, P.A. Gerber, M. Pollet, K.M. Rolfes, A.A. Soshilov, M.S. Denison, A.A. Momin, S.T. Arold, A. Datsi, S.A. Braun, P. Oláh, M.E. Lacouture, J. Krutmann, T. Haarmann-Stemmann, B. Homey, S. Meller, Vemurafenib acts as an aryl hydrocarbon receptor antagonist: Implications for inflammatory cutaneous adverse events, Allergy. 74 (2019) 2437-2448. doi:10.1111/all.13972.

[48] J.H. Hwang, K. Kannan, T.J. Evans, H. Iwata, E.Y. Kim, Assessment of Risks of Dioxins for Aryl Hydrocarbon Receptor-Mediated Effects in Polar Bear (Ursus maritimus) by in Vitro and in Silico Approaches, Environ. Sci. Technol. 54 (2020) 1770-1781. doi:10.1021/acs.est.9b05941.

[49] K.N. Chitrala, X. Yang, P. Nagarkatti, M. Nagarkatti, Comparative analysis of interactions between aryl hydrocarbon receptor ligand binding domain with its ligands: A computational study, BMC Struct. Biol. 18 (2018) 1-17. doi:10.1186/s12900-018-0095-2.

[50] P. Ramadoss, G.H. Perdew, Use of 2-azido-3-[125I]iodo-7,8-dibromodibenzo-p-dioxin as a probe to determine the relative ligand affinity of human versus mouse aryl hydrocarbon receptor in cultured cells, Mol. Pharmacol. 66 (2004) 129-136. doi:10.1124/mol.66.1.129.

[51] C. Odio, S.A. Holzman, M.S. Denison, D. Fraccalvieri, L. Bonati, D.G. Franks, M.E. Hahn, W.H. Powell, Specific ligand binding domain residues confer low dioxin responsiveness to AHR1β of xenopus laevis, Biochemistry.

52 (2013) 1746-1754. doi:10.1021/bi301722k.

[52] A. Pandini, A.A. Soshilov, Y. Song, J. Zhao, L. Bonati, M.S. Denison, Detection of the TCDD binding-fingerprint within the Ah receptor ligand binding domain by structurally driven mutagenesis and functional analysis, Biochemistry. 48 (2009) 5972-5983. doi:10.1021/bi900259z.

[53] M.S. Denison, A.A. Soshilov, G. He, D.E. Degroot, B. Zhao, Exactly the same but different: Promiscuity and diversity in the molecular mechanisms of action of the aryl hydrocarbon (dioxin) receptor, Toxicol. Sci. 124 (2011) 1-22. doi:10.1093/toxsci/kfr218.

[54] I. Motto, A. Bordogna, A.A. Soshilov, M.S. Denison, L. Bonati, New aryl hydrocarbon receptor homology model targeted to improve docking reliability, J. Chem. Inf. Model. 51 (2011) 2868-2881. doi:10.1021/ci2001617.

[55] S. Miyagi, K. Murata, K. Sashino, S. Sawamura, S. Uruno, S. Yoshimura, E. Akahoshi, M. Ishihara-Sugano, S. Itoh, N. Kurita, Binding affinity between AhR and exogenous/endogenous ligands: Molecular simulations and biological experiment, Mol. Simul. 41 (2015) 555-563. doi:10.1080/08927022.2014.899696.

[56] M. Kumar Gadhwal, S. Patil, P. D'mello, A. Joshi, Homology modeling of aryl hydrocarbon receptor and docking of agonists and antagonists, n.d.

[57] A. Pandini, M.S. Denison, Y. Song, A.A. Soshilov, L. Bonati, Structural and functional characterization of the aryl hydrocarbon receptor ligand binding domain by homology modeling and mutational analysis, Biochemistry. 46 (2007) 696-708. doi:10.1021/bi061460t.

[58] A.A. Soshilov, M.S. Denison, Ligand Promiscuity of Aryl Hydrocarbon Receptor Agonists and Antagonists Revealed by Site-Directed Mutagenesis, Mol. Cell. Biol. 34 (2014) 1707-1719. doi:10.1128/mcb.01183-13.

[59] C. Knebel, J. Kebben, I. Eberini, L. Palazzolo, H.S. Hammer, R.D. Süssmuth, T. Heise, S. Hessel-Pras, A. Lampen, A. Braeuning, P. Marx-Stoelting, Propiconazole is an activator of AHR and causes concentration additive effects with an established AHR ligand, Arch. Toxicol. 92 (2018) 3471-3486. doi:10.1007/s00204-018-2321-x.

[60] W.H. Bisson, D.C. Koch, E.F. O'Donnell, S.M. Khalil, N.I. Kerkvliet, R.L. Tanguay, R. Abagyan, S.K. Kolluri, Modeling of the aryl hydrocarbon receptor (AhR) ligand binding domain and its utility in virtual ligand screening to predict new AhR ligands, J. Med. Chem. 52 (2009) 5635-5641. doi:10.1021/jm900199u.

[61] J.-H. Hwang, S. Bak, E.-Y. Kim, In Silico Analysis of the Interaction of Avian Aryl Hydrocarbon Receptors and Dioxins to Decipher Isoform-, Ligand-, and Species-Specific Activations, Artic. Environ. Sci. Technol. 49 (2015) 3795-3804. doi:10.1021/es505733f.

[62] B. Wu, Y. Zhang, J. Kong, X. Zhang, S. Cheng, In silico predication of nuclear hormone receptors for organic pollutants by homology modeling and molecular docking, Toxicol. Lett. 191 (2009) 69-73. doi:10.1016/j.toxlet.2009.08.005.

[63] Ž. Jakopin, Assessment of the endocrine-disrupting potential of halogenated parabens: An in silico approach, Chemosphere. 264 (2021) 128447. doi:10.1016/j.chemosphere.2020.128447.

[64] X. Gao, C. Xie, Y. Wang, Y. Luo, T. Yagai, D. Sun, X. Qin, K.W. Krausz, F.J. Gonzalez, The antiandrogen flutamide is a novel aryl hydrocarbon receptor ligand that disrupts bile acid

homeostasis in mice through induction of Abcc 4, Biochem. Pharmacol. 119 (2016) 93-104. doi:10.1016/j.bcp.2016.08.021.

[65] D. Corrada, A.A. Soshilov, M.S. Denison, L. Bonati, Deciphering Dimerization Modes of PAS Domains: Computational and Experimental Analyses of the AhR:ARNT Complex Reveal New Insights Into the Mechanisms of AhR Transformation, PLOS Comput. Biol. 12 (2016) e1004981. doi:10.1371/journal.pcbi.1004981.

[66] T. Zhu, S. Cao, P.C. Su, R. Patel, D. Shah, H.B. Chokshi, R. Szukala, M.E. Johnson, K.E. Hevener, Hit identification and optimization in virtual screening: Practical recommendations based on a critical literature analysis, J. Med. Chem. 56 (2013) 6560-6572. doi:10.1021/jm301916b.

[67] J. Vázquez, M. López, E. Gibert, E. Herrero, F. Javier Luque, Merging ligand-based and structure-based methods in drug discovery: an overview of combined virtual screening approaches, Molecules. 25 (2020) 4723. doi:10.3390/molecules25204723.

[68] C. Acharya, A. Coop, J. E. Polli, A. D. Mac Kerell, Recent Advances in Ligand-Based Drug Design: Relevance and Utility of the Conformationally Sampled Pharmacophore Approach, Curr. Comput. Aided-Drug Des. 7 (2010) 10-22. doi:10.2174/1573 40911793743547.

[69] S.U. Khan, N. Ahemad, L.H. Chuah, R. Naidu, T.T. Htar, Sequential ligand- and structure-based virtual screening approach for the identification of potential G protein-coupled estrogen receptor-1 (GPER-1) modulators, RSC Adv. 9 (2019) 2525-2538. doi:10.1039/c8ra09318k.

[70] X. Qing, X.Y. Lee, J. De Raeymaeker, J.R. Tame, K.Y. Zhang, M. De Maeyer, A.R. Voet, Video abstract Pharmacophore modeling: advances, limitations, and current utility in drug discovery, J. Receptor. Ligand Channel Res. 16 (2021). doi:10.2147/JRLCR.S46843.

[71] Z. Wang, H. Sun, C. Shen, X. Hu, J. Gao, D. Li, D. Cao, T. Hou, Combined strategies in structure-based virtual screening, Phys. Chem. Chem. Phys. 22 (2020) 3149-3159. doi:10.1039/c9cp06303j.

[72] M. Wieder, A. Garon, U. Perricone, S. Boresch, T. Seidel, A.M. Almerico, T. Langer, Common Hits Approach: Combining Pharmacophore Modeling and Molecular Dynamics Simulations, J. Chem. Inf. Model. 57 (2017) 365-385. doi:10.1021/acs.jcim.6b00674.

[73] S. Debnath, T. Debnath, S. Bhaumik, S. Majumdar, A.M. Kalle, V. Aparna, Discovery of novel potential selective HDAC8 inhibitors by combine ligand-based, structure-based virtual screening and in-vitro biological evaluation, Sci. Rep. 9 (2019) 1-14. doi:10.1038/s41598-019-53376-y.

[74] V.K. Gupta, P.S. Rana, Toxicity prediction of small drug molecules of aryl hydrocarbon receptor using a proposed ensemble model, Turkish J. Electr. Eng. Comput. Sci. 27 (2019) 2833-2849. doi:10.3906/elk-1809-9.

[75] H. Xiao, N. Mei, Q. Chi, X. Wang, Comprehensive binding analysis of polybrominated diphenyl ethers and aryl hydrocarbon receptor via an integrated molecular modeling approach, Chemosphere. 262 (2021) 128356. doi:10.1016/j.chemosphere.2020.128356.

[76] A.L.W. Po, W. Zhang, What lessons can be learnt from withdrawal of mibefradil from the market?, Lancet. 351 (1998) 1829-1830. doi:10.1016/S0140-6736(05)78800-0.

[77] S.N. Rath, L. Jena, M. Patri, Understanding ligands driven mechanism of wild and mutant aryl hydrocarbon receptor in presence of phytochemicals combating Parkinson's disease: an in silico and in vivo study, J. Biomol. Struct. Dyn. 38 (2020) 807-826. doi:10.1080/07391102.2019.1590240.

[78] Y. Matsuzaka, T. Hosaka, A. Ogaito, K. Yoshinari, Y. Uesawa, Prediction Model of Aryl Hydrocarbon Receptor Activation by a Novel QSAR Approach, Deep Snap–Deep Learning, Molecules. 25 (2020) 1317. doi:10.3390/molecules25061317.

[79] K. Zhu, C. Shen, C. Tang, Y. Zhou, C. He, Z. Zuo, Improvement in the screening performance of potential aryl hydrocarbon receptor ligands by using supervised machine learning, Chemosphere. 265 (2021) 129099. doi:10.1016/j.chemosphere.2020.129099.

[80] E. Goya-Jorge, R.M. Giner, M. Sylla-Iyarreta Veitía, R. Gozalbes, S.J. Barigye, Predictive modeling of aryl hydrocarbon receptor (AhR) agonism, Chemosphere. 256 (2020) 127068. doi:10.1016/j.chemosphere.2020.127068.

[81] Z. Ek Dvo R Ak, K. Poulíkov, S. Mani, Indole scaffolds as a promising class of the aryl hydrocarbon receptor ligands, (2021). doi:10.1016/j.ejmech.2021.113231.

[82] A. Tkachenko, F. Henkler, J. Brinkmann, J. Sowada, D. Genkinger, C. Kern, T. Tralau, A. Luch, The Q-rich/PST domain of the AHR regulates both ligand-induced nuclear transport and nucleocytoplasmic shuttling, Sci. Rep. 6 (2016) 1-11. doi:10.1038/srep32009.

Chapter 6

Developing a Novel Multiplexed Immune Assay Platform to Screen Kinase Modulators of T Cell Activation

Zhaoping Liu, Andrea Gomez-Donart, Caroline Weldon, Nina Senutovitch and John O'Rourke

Abstract

T cell activation plays a central role in inflammation, autoimmune diseases and cancer. Cancer immunotherapies, such as immune checkpoint inhibitor, bi-specific antibody, chimeric antigen receptor T (CAR T) cell, and adoptive tumor-infiltrating lymphocyte (TIL) therapies require the characterization and monitoring of T cell activation. Here we describe a novel, multiplex immune assay platform based on high-throughput flow cytometry technology and advanced computational algorithms for data analysis. The assay simultaneously measures T cell dynamics including phenotype, time-dependent expression of activation markers, secreted effector cytokines, and proliferation. The assay screened a kinase chemogenomic library and identified 25 kinase inhibitors with distinct inhibition profiles on early (CD69) and late (CD25) activation markers and the cytokines IFNγ and TNFα. We identified 5 kinase inhibitors with dissimilar effects on CD69 and CD25 expression, and a cluster of total 4 MEK1//2 inhibitors with similar activation profiles. The screening revealed 3 kinase inhibitors for PKC, IKK2, and MEK1/2 respectively, all with a phenotypic signature similar to ruxolitinib, a Jak1/2 inhibitor used to treat myelofibrosis disease. These results suggest this multiplexed assay platform, combined with a chemogenomic library screening, may be used as primary screen for phenotypic or target-based drug discovery, target identification, and potential drug repositioning.

Keywords: T cell activation, high-throughput screening, flow cytometry, kinase inhibitor, drug repositioning

1. Introduction

Unraveling the complex biochemistry of the immune system in search of innovative therapies is a new frontier of drug discovery with hundreds of autoimmune disease therapies and thousands of immuno-oncology therapies in the global development pipeline [1, 2].

Hallmarks of autoimmune disease pathogenesis are abnormal CD4 and CD8 T cell activation [3]. Genetic defects, mutations and other mechanisms resulting in increased T cell activity are involved in many autoimmune pathologies making them attractive targets for the direct inhibition of T cell activation [4]. T helper cells —characterized by the expression of the surface molecule CD4—release cytokines that shape the immune response and pathology in autoimmune and inflammatory diseases [5].

Cancer immunotherapies are moving to the forefront of cancer treatment with a variety of regimens, such as immune checkpoint blockade therapies targeting T cells' regulatory pathways to enhance T cell activation and its anti-tumor immune responses. Focusing on immune checkpoint inhibitors is a disruptive change in immuno-oncology. Rather than directly attacking the tumor cell itself, the checkpoint inhibition strategy is removing inhibitory pathways by targeting the molecules involved in T cell regulation that block effective anti-tumor responses [6]. Another type of cancer immunotherapy consists of bispecific antibodies designed to redirect immune cells to tumor sites where they induce immune synapse formation, immune cell activation, cytokine secretion and proliferation leading to tumor lysis [7].

The versatile T cell weapon can also be deployed directly via adoptive T cell transfer (ACT). ACT involves infusion of in vitro expanded antigen-specific lymphocytes such as chimeric antigen receptor T (CAR-T) cells or tumor infiltrating lymphocytes (TILs) to cancer patients to mediate antitumor effects [8–10]. The T cell-mediated tumor cell killing is through tumor antigen recognition, robust T cell activation, proliferation and in vivo cytotoxicity. Different types of cancer immunotherapies can be combined or given sequentially to further enhance the magnitude of antitumor immune response over single agents [11].

In the adaptive immune response, the binding of the T cell receptor to peptides complexed with the major histocompatibility complex (MHC) on antigen-presenting cells, along with engagement of co-receptors such as CD4 or CD8 and co-stimulatory molecules such as CD28, triggers an intricate signal cascade. The key to T cell-mediated immune responses are the multiple intracellular biochemical events involving the complex interaction of cytosolic tyrosine kinases and serine–threonine kinases [12]. Kinases as drug targets have been investigated for decades in autoimmune disease, cancer, and degenerative diseases [13]. The kinase signaling pathway through Raf/MEK/ERK1/2 is a major regulator of cell proliferation and survival, and hyper-activation of this pathway is associated with human tumor malignancies [14]. Currently 37 kinase inhibitors have received FDA approval for treatment of malignancies such as breast and lung cancer. There are 150 kinase-targeted drugs in clinical trials, and kinase-specific inhibitors are in the preclinical stage of drug development [15]. In addition, combinations of kinase inhibitors are being explored for the treatment of cancer, and preclinical and clinical data demonstrate that therapeutic combinations enhance primary antitumor responses and delay the onset of resistance [16]. Kinase signaling also regulates the immune system and modulates the tumor immune microenvironment. Inhibition of kinase activity such as phosphoinositide 3-kinase (PI3K) promotes anti-tumor immunity through direct enhancement of CD8+ T cell activation and suppression of T regulatory cells [17]. The combination of kinase inhibition with cancer immunotherapy is another emerging research area as demonstrated in recent preclinical studies that showed the kinase inhibitor of P21 Activated Kinase 4 (PAK4) boosted PD-1 therapy in animal models [18].

Whether it is the characterization of immune phenotype or function, or the screening or profiling of biological or small molecule drug candidates, high-throughput flow cytometry and its ability to perform multi-parametric analyses of single cells or particles is playing an increasingly pivotal role in quantifying the myriad aspects of drug discovery [19, 20]. Here we developed a novel, multiplexed T cell activation assay platform based on high-throughput flow cytometry and associated advanced data analysis algorithms. As a proof-of concept, we screened a kinase chemogenomic compound library and identified kinase inhibitors with various inhibition profiles of T cell activation, monitored by sampling a small aliquot from a mixture of cells and beads in a microtiter plate.

2. Materials and methods

2.1 Cell lines and reagents

The kinase inhibitor library (Cayman, Cat#10505) used for the screening assay has 152 known kinase inhibitors at 10 mM stock concentration in DMSO. The fluorescent antibodies against CD3, CD4, CD8, CD69, CD25 and HLA-DR, cell viability dye, cell proliferation tracing dye, cytokine capture beads (iQue QBeads®, Sartorius) and the cytokine detection reagents used in this study are from the iQue® Human T Cell Activation Kit (iQue® Sartorius, Cat#90561). Human PBMCs (Astarte Biologics, Cat#1001) from healthy donors were stimulated/activated with either T-activator CD3/CD28 Dynabeads® (ThermoFisher, Cat#11131D) or phytohemagglutinin (PHA, Sigma, Cat#L8754), or Enterotoxin Type B from *Staphylococcus aureus* (SEB, List Biological Laboratories, Cat#122). Cells were cultured in RMPI-1640 (VWR, Cat#45000–396) with 10% fetal bovine serum (VWR, Cat#97068–085) and supplements that included non-essential amino acids (VWR, Cat#12001–634), sodium pyruvate (VWR, Cat#45000–710), and penicillin–streptomycin (VWR, Cat#12001–692).

2.2 Assay development and characterization

2.2.1 Day-to-day profiling of T cell activation

The assay was run using cryopreserved human PBMCs from a single healthy donor and were allowed to recover for 24 hours before use. On day 0, we stained human PBMCs with cell proliferation tracing dye (excitation: 488 nm and emission: 530/30 nm) and washed 3 times before plating into a 96-well plate at 2 million/mL (50 μL/well). We treated the cells by adding 50 μL/well of 3 different T-cell modulators in the respective wells: CD3/CD28 Dynabeads, PHA, or SEB. We performed an 11-point, 1:2 serial titration with duplicate wells per dose for each selected treatment. The final top concentration of the treatment in the assay well was 1 million/mL CD3/CD28 Dynabeads, 10 μg/mL PHA, or 100 ng/mL SEB, respectively. The untreated wells (with a concentration of zero) were used as negative controls for each treatment. On each day of culture (days 1, 3, and 6), we mixed the cell/supernatant sample in the culture plate by manual pipetting up and down 8 times. We transferred 10 μL cell/supernatant sample per well without dilution from the culture plate to a 96-well assay plate (Costar, Cat#3897), and stained the samples following the iQue® Human T Cell Activation Kit assay protocol. In the assay plate, 2 rows of wells (rows A and B) were designated for standard curve generation with a mixture of 2 protein standards (IFNγ and TNFα) in each well. Top concentration was 50,000 pg./mL for each protein in the standard mixture with 1:3 serial titration and duplicate wells per concentration. The lowest concentration was set to zero to determine background. Rows C-H were assigned to samples from 3 different treatment regimens: CD3/CD28 Dynabeads, PHA or SEB (**Supplemental Figure 1**). After staining and washing, samples from the full plate were acquired in approximately 15 minutes using the iQue® Screener PLUS (Sartorius), a high-throughput flow cytometry platform which has violet, blue and red lasers, and a total of 13 fluorescent channels. In each sample well of the assay plates, levels of secreted cytokines (IFNγ and TNFα) were interpolated by reference to the corresponding standard curves generated from the standard wells in the same assay plate.

2.2.2 Z' factor characterization of T cell activation

The Z' factor of the assay was calculated to evaluate assay variation. The study was run similarly to the day-to-day profiling study described earlier, with minor modification. Cryopreserved human PBMCs from a single healthy donor were allowed to recover for 24 hours before use. On day 0 we plated the recovered PBMCs into a 96-well plate at 2 million/mL (50 μL/well). Then, we treated the cells by adding the same volume of CD3/CD28 Dynabeads. Total volume per well was 100 μL at the final concentration, with a total of 3 plates run. In each culture plate there were 24 wells without Dynabeads (negative control), and 24 treated wells with CD3/CD28 Dynabeads (positive control) with a final bead density of 1 million/mL. After culturing 24, 48, or 72-hours, we mixed the cell/supernatant samples in the culture plate by manual pipetting 8 times. We transferred 10 μL of cell/supernatant sample per well without dilution, from the culture plates to 96-well assay plates and stained following the iQue® Human T Cell Activation Kit assay protocol. After staining and washing, samples from each plate were acquired on the iQue® Screener PLUS. iQue Forecyt® software was used to perform Z'-Factor plate calculations on well data of the positive and negative controls. For each plate, a single Z'-Factor was calculated as follows [Eq. 1]:

$$Z-factor = 1 - \frac{3(\sigma_p + \sigma_n)}{|\mu_p + \mu_n|} \qquad (1)$$

- σ_p = standard deviation of the positive control wells for each plate
- σ_n = standard deviation of the negative control wells for each plate
- μ_p = mean of the positive control wells for each plate
- μ_n = mean of the negative control wells for each plate

Positive control wells: CD3/CD28 Dynabeads-treated wells with bead/cell ratio at 1:1. Both Dynabeads and PBMC concentrations were at 1 million/mL. Negative control wells: cells only without CD3/CD28 Dynabeads.

2.3 Kinase inhibitors screening

2.3.1 Culture setup for screening

The cryopreserved PBMCs from a single healthy donor were allowed to recover for 24 hours before use. On day 0 we plated the recovered PBMCs into a 96-well plate at 4 million/mL (25 μL/well). We then added 25 μL of 40 μM kinase inhibitors (in culture media) into each well with cells to reach 20 μM inhibitor concentration. The negative control was culture media only and the positive control was 20 μM cyclosporine A. We mixed the culture and incubated for 1 hour with 5% CO_2 at 37° C. We then added 50 μL (2 million/mL) of CD3/CD28 Dynabeads into each well of the screening culture plate. The final cell and Dynabead density were 1 million/mL each, and the final kinase inhibitor concentration was 10 μM. After mixing, the culture plate was incubated for 24 hours with 5% CO_2 at 37°C.

2.3.2 The screening assay

The screening assay was performed after a 24-hour treatment. Because all wells of the 2 screening plates were filled with the kinase inhibitors and controls, we used a third plate for the standard curve generation. For the standard curve plate, only the top 2 rows were used. Top concentration for each standard in the mixture was 50,000 pg./mL, with a 1:3 serial titration and duplicate wells. The lowest concentration was zero for negative control purposes. After a 24-hour culture for the 2 screening culture plates, we mixed the cell/supernatant samples in the culture plates by manual pipetting up and down 8 times and then transferred 10 μL of the cell/supernatant sample per well, without dilution from the 2 culture plates to the 2 screening assay plates. We stained the plates following the iQue® Human T Cell Activation Kit assay protocol. After staining and washing, the samples from each plate were acquired on the iQue® Screener PLUS. After data acquisition, the secreted levels of 2 cytokines (IFNγ and TNFα) in the 2 screening plates were interpolated using the iQue Forecyt® software by referring to the corresponding standard curves generated from the standard-only plate.

2.3.3 Dosage test of kinase inhibitors

After screening the kinase inhibitor library, we selected some compounds for further characterization by dosage testing. The test workflow was the same as the screening workflow described earlier with the exception of a series of kinase inhibitor concentrations. We performed 11-point, 1:2 serial titration with duplicate wells per dose for each selected compound. The final top concentration in the assay well was 10 μM for each selected compound. The concentration at zero μM was used as negative control (background) for each compound.

2.3.4 General data acquisition and analysis method

The iQue® Human T Cell Activation Kit comes with a template with predefined gates. Other analytical functions, such as heat maps, are queued to automatically populate. During data acquisition, events populated in the dot plots within the templated gates. The iQue QBeads® (for cytokine quantitation) and the cells were segregated based on size. Singlet beads were gated in a 2D plot of forward scatter (FSC)-height vs. FSC-area. After data acquisition on the iQue® Screener PLUS, all the cell and bead populations of interest were gated at the plate level. As shown in **Figure 1B**, the gating strategy separates cytokine capture beads from PBMC cells in an FSC vs. side scatter (SSC) plot, based on size and granularity differences. Singlet beads were gated in an FSC-height vs. FSC-area, and 2 different cytokine capture beads (iQue QBeads®) were separated in an RL1 (excitation: 640 nm; emission: 675/30 nm) vs. RL2 (excitation: 640 nm; emission: 780/60 nm) plot. Singlet cells are gated in an FSC-height vs. FSC-area plot. Live cells were gated in an RL1 vs. SSC plot. In live cell population, proliferated cells (dim fluorescent population) were gated from non-proliferated cells (bright fluorescent population) by using an overlay BL1 (excitation: 488 nm; emission: 530/30 nm) 1D histogram with positive and negative controls (data not shown). Also, from the live cell population, CD3+ T cells were separated from non-T cells in a CD3 vs. SSC plot. CD4+ T helper cells were separated from CD8 T cytotoxic cells in a CD4 vs. CD8 plot. CD69+, CD25+ and HLA-DR+ CD4 or CD8 T cells were gated in the corresponding plots with the markers at x-axis and SSC at y-axis. iQue Forecyt® software generated the standard curves (IFNγ and TNFα) using a 4-parameter logistic (4PL) regression fit with $1/Y^2$

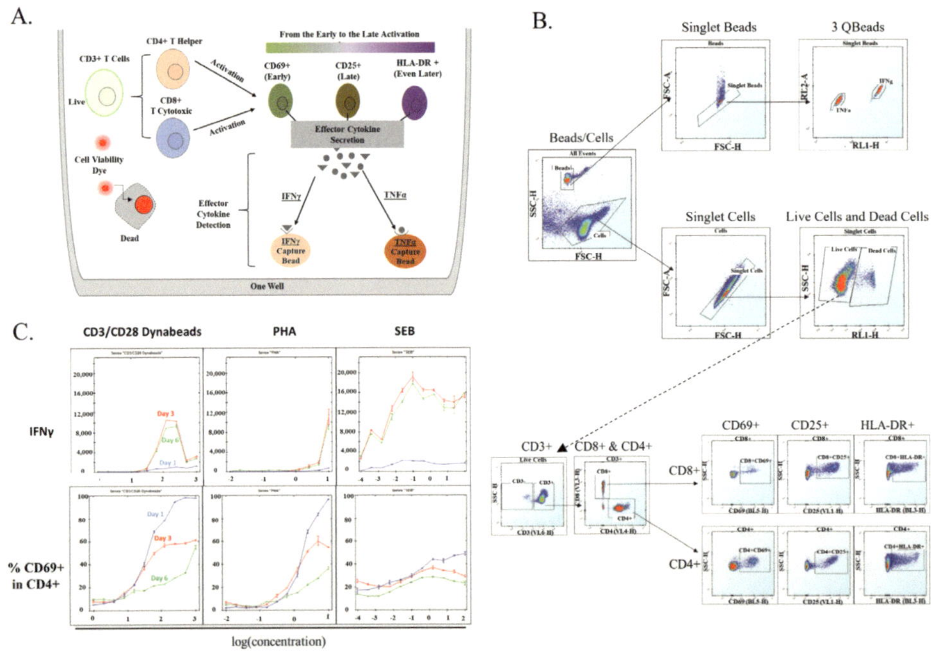

Figure 1.
Develop a multiplexed T cell activation assay. (A) a novel multiplexed T cell activation assay in a cell and bead mixture format. T cells in each assay well are stained with cell viability dye to differentiate live cells and dead cells. Cells are stained with CD3, CD4 and CD8 fluorescent antibodies to identify the CD4+ T helper cells and CD8+ T cytotoxic cells. Different T cell activation status is analyzed by staining with cell surface markers: CD69 (early activation marker), CD25 (late activation markers), and HLA-DR (even later activation markers). In the same assay well, the secreted IFNγ and TNFα after T cell activation are simultaneously measured by 2 cytokine capture beads in a sandwich immunoassay format. (B) the gating strategy for digital separation of the cytokine beads and the activated T cells acquired by high-throughput flow cytometry. After the sample from each well is acquired by iQue® screener PLUS, the cell/bead events are analyzed by iQue Forecyt® software (Sartorius), and cells and beads can be separated, based on the size and granularity, in FSC/SSC plot. IFNγ and TNFα capture beads are separated, based on the different bead intrinsic fluorescence in red fluorescence channels (RL1 and RL2 with excitation both at 640 nm, and with emission 675/30 nm and 780/60 nm, respectively). For cell phenotyping gating, live cells are separated from dead cells which are brightly stained by the cell viability dye intercalated with DNA. Live cells can be separated to CD3+ T cells and CD3- non-T cells. Based on CD4 and CD8 expression level, CD4+ T helper cells and CD8+ T cytotoxic cells are separated for further identification of early activation (CD69+), late activation (CD25+) and even later activation (HLA-DR+). (C) Representative data of time dependent profiling of 3 different modulators of T cell activation assay. 3 different modulators (CD3/CD28 Dynabeads, PHA and SEB) showed distinct signature of dose-dependent and time-dependent IFNγ secretion and the expression of early activation marker CD69. The unit is k/mL for CD3/CD28 Dynabeads, µg/mL for PHA, and ng/mL for SEB. Each data point represents mean ± standard deviation (n = 2 wells).

weighting factor. The linear range for each standard curve was generated automatically using iQue Forecyt® software with the following equations:

$$Y_{Bend\ Lower} = \frac{(a-d)}{\frac{(1+1)}{k}} + d \qquad (2)$$

$$Y_{Bend\ Higher} = \frac{(a-d)}{(1+k)} + d \qquad (3)$$

$$X_{Bend} = c\left(\frac{a - Y_{bend}}{Y_{bend-d}}\right)^\wedge \frac{1}{b} \qquad (4)$$

- Y is the response
- X is the concentration

- a is the lower asymptote
- b is slope
- c is EC_{50}
- d is the upper asymptote
- k is a constant equal to 4.6805

Each cytokine concentration was interpolated by reference in the iQue Forecyt® software to the corresponding cytokine standard curve generated from the same assay plate, or from the standard-only plate.

2.3.5 Algorithms used for hit identification

We used a multi-plate analysis algorithm in the iQue Forecyt® software and a function called Profile Map based on Boolean logic to identify hits in the screening that simultaneously met multiple specified criteria across multiple plates. The hits were also ranked and compared in a line graph.

3. Results

3.1 Assay characterization

The goal of assay characterization was to evaluate assay robustness, verify the ability to differentiate the modulators of T cell activation, and determine if the assay would require optimization to screen a chemogenomic kinase library.

The assay was designed to achieve a wide dynamic range to detect high levels of these cytokines: IFNγ, linear range 91–22,204 pg./mL and TNFα, linear range 181–50,000 pg./mL. The detection range is even wider than the linear range (data not shown). This wide dynamic range ensures the detection of high levels of secreted IFNγ and TNFα after T cell activation and eliminates a sample dilution step.

The assay variation was characterized and analyzed by measuring the Z' factor of 24-hour T cell activation with CD3/CD28 Dynabeads as a positive control and with untreated sample as a negative control. The mean Z' factor is 0.8 for both the percentage of CD69+ cells in CD4+ cells and for the percentage of CD69+ in CD8+ cells; 0.9 for both the percentage of CD25+ in CD4+ and for the percentage of CD25 + in CD8+ cells; −0.1 and 0.2 for the percentage of HLA-DR+ in CD4+ and CD8+ cells, respectively; 0.4 (IFNγ), and 0.7 (TNFα). As expected, a very low Z' factor for HLA-DR endpoint is a result of the late expression of this molecule after T cell activation. Forty-eight-hour and 72-hour activation did achieve higher HLA-DR Z' factor (0.3–0.5) than 24-hour activation. Different T cell activation timing may impact the signal of each endpoint and then, correspondingly, change the Z' factors. The Z' factors of 0.5 or higher in a multiplexed cell/bead-based mixture assay, suggest that the assay variation is appropriate for screening.

In order to evaluate the assay robustness in differentiating various compounds over different treatment time, we ran a day-to-day test monitoring of T cell activation. **Figure 1** shows the assay biochemistry (**Figure 1A**), and the cell/beads gating strategy (**Figure 1B**). **Figure 1C** of the day-to-day profiling results with 3 modulators demonstrated the assay robustness as a proof of concept. Only IFNγ and CD69+ cell endpoints are shown as examples. The results showed the 3 different modulators had distinct profiles in IFNγ secretion, and in the expression of the early activation marker CD69. In addition, the results displayed a day-to-day effect. For the CD3/CD28 Dynabeads-treated condition, day 1 showed a dose-dependent IFNγ secretion, and day 3 and day 6 showed similar IFNγ secretion and saturation at a relatively high concentration. Even more interesting, the top 2 doses on day 3 and day 6 showed reduced IFNγ secretion ("hook" effect), which was consistent with the T cell exhaustion phenomenon characteristic of T cell activation [21]. Other endpoints also achieved distinct profiles including T cell proliferation determined by using a proliferation dye (data not shown).

3.2 General screening results

As shown in **Supplement Figure 1**, screening the kinase inhibitor library (Cayman 152 kinase inhibitors) involved two assay screening plates.

Screening results of the kinase inhibitors on CD69 expression are shown in **Figure 2**, an iQue Forecyt® visualization function that displays a thumbnail dot plot of each well on the plate. This example shows a CD69 vs. SSC 2D plot. The figure shows only the first screening plate with CD4+ T cells as an example. Wells highlighted in bright red boxes, as examples in **Figure 2A**, show various inhibition of CD69 expression by inhibitors of 5 different kinase classes. **Figure 2B** shows a

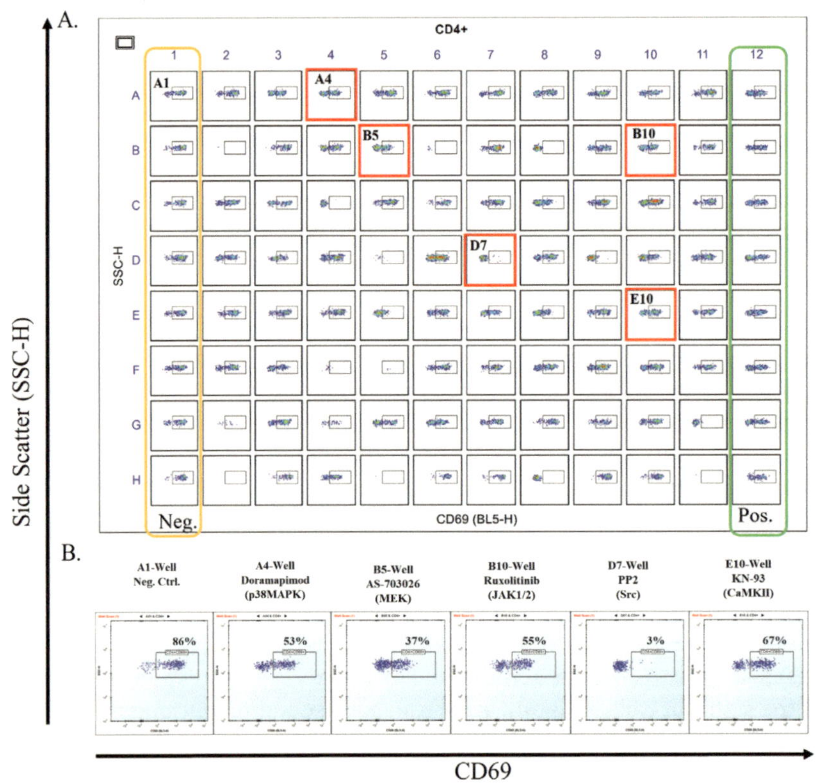

Figure 2.
The representative screening results: Kinase inhibitors decrease the expression of the early activation marker CD69 on CD4+ T helper cells in the plate 1. (A) the plate view of 2D plots (CD69 vs. SSC) that showed the CD69 expression in each well. Five screening wells with decreasing CD69 expression, as examples, were highlighted with red boxes. (B) the well-based 2D plots (CD69 vs. SSC) from five highlighted wells and a negative control well (A1 well) showed different decrease of early activation marker CD69 induced by different kinase inhibitors.

zoomed-in view of each well highlighted in red and a negative control well (A1). The results suggest the assay can pick out different compounds as hits from different classes of kinase inhibitors.

To identify hits from the screen that meet multiple criteria, we used the iQue Forecyt® multi-plate and Profile Map algorithms to distinguish hits by dialing in the exact characteristics from multiple criteria. **Figure 3A** shows the 11 thresholds used to identify hits that decrease the cytokine secretion and the expression of these cell surface activation markers: IFNγ concentration, TNFα concentration, cell viability (Live Cells as % of total cells), CD4+ CD69+ as % of CD4+, CD8 + CD69+ as % of CD8+, CD4+ CD25+ as % of CD4, CD8+ CD25+ as % of CD8, CD4+ HLA-DR+ as % of CD4+, CD8+ HLA-DR+ as % of CD8+, Count of CD4+, Count of CD8+. HLA-DR was not critical in the criteria mix because it is a very late activation marker and is not highly expressed after 24 hours of activation. **Figure 3B** shows the wells (in blue) that meet the criteria specified in the iQue Forecyt® Profile Map. The positive control (cyclosporine A) is excluded from analysis (**Figure 3B**, column 12 on both plates) so that hits from only the samples can be generated for hit ranking (**Figure 3C**). The ranking is based on % CD69+ in CD4+ (from low to high). The IFNγ and TNFα level was normalized against the negative control as expressed at percentage (to fit into the same scale). A total of 25 hits showed broad inhibition of all major T cell activation markers including CD69, CD25, IFNγ, and TNFα. Interestingly, some patterns showed strong inhibition of cytokine secretion

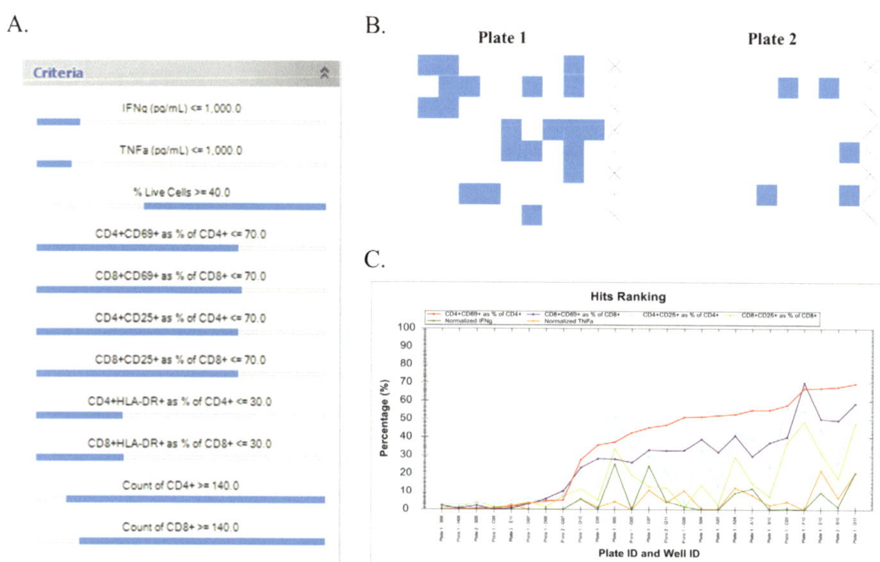

Figure 3.
The identification and ranking of the screening hits that inhibit broadly the secreted cytokine and the expression of the cell surface activation markers. Data were analyzed by iQue Forecyt® software's multi-plate analysis and profile map tools (Sartorius). (A) the 11 criteria used to identify the screening hits. All 11 criteria were applied simultaneously to help identify the screening hits. The criteria are subjective, based on these general concepts: Inhibition of T cell activation will decrease cytokine secretion and expression of cell surface activation markers; the "hit well" should have a pre-determined number of viable T cells; and, the desired percentage of hits. (B) the profile maps of two screening plates with a total of 25 screening hits (see blue boxes). The negative control, column 1 on both plates did not show hits as expected. Column 12 (positive controls) on both plates, which did show as positive (data not shown), were excluded from analysis for the hit ranking purpose. (C) the 25 screening hits out 152 kinase inhibitors from the whole library were ranked, based on the decrease (from low to high) of CD69 expression on CD4+ T cells (red curve) by using line graph feature in iQue Forecyt®. Other parameters were also shown for the 25 hits, including CD69 expression in CD8+ T cytotoxic cells, CD25 expression in CD4+ T helper and in CD8+ T cytotoxic cells, the normalized secretion of IFNγ and TNFα (normalized to the mean value of the negative wells, as expressed by the percentage).

but medium inhibition of cell surface activation markers, while some compounds strongly inhibit almost every activation marker.

3.3 Identification of compounds with distinct activation profiles

Using the multi-plate analysis algorithm and Profile Map Boolean logic algorithm in the iQue Forecyt® software we identified 2 compounds, tunicamycin and an erbastatin analog, that have no, or very moderate, effect on CD69+ while having medium to strong inhibition on CD25 and IFNγ and TNFα (**Figure 4**). Tunicamycin

A.

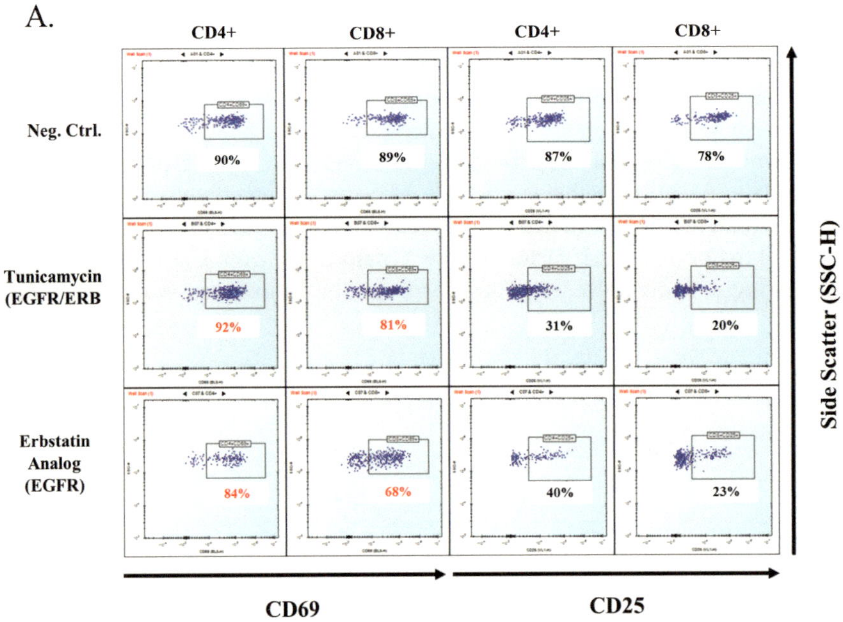

B.

	IFNγ (pg/mL)	TNFα (pg/mL)
Neg. Ctrl.	3,915	3,157
Tunicamycin (EGFR/ERB)	21	719
Erbstatin Analog (EGFR)	228	422

C.

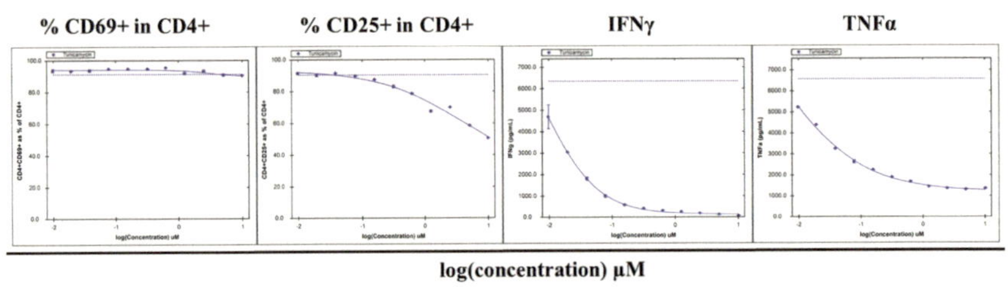

Figure 4.
Kinase inhibitors that barely decreased early activation marker CD69 but did inhibit the expression of the late activation marker CD25 and did decrease the secreted IFNγ and TNFα. (A) 2D plots (CD69 or CD25 vs. SSC) from the screening wells of these 2 inhibitors and the negative control well showed less effect on CD69 expression (see the red numbers) but with drastic decreasing effect on CD25 expression on both CD4+ T helper cells and CD8+ T cytotoxic cells. (B) Table showing the compounds Tunicamycin (EGFR/ERB inhibitor) and an erbstatin analog (EGFR inhibitor) had the significant decreasing effect on the secretion of IFNγ and TNFα. (C) Example of tunicamycin's effect, from a separate dosage test experiment, on the decreasing of other markers except CD69 expression. Each point in the graph represent the mean ± standard deviation of the duplicate wells. The dash line in each graph shows the baseline level without the compound.

decreases CD69+ cells in CD4+ and CD8+ cells −2% and 8%, respectively, but significantly decreases CD25+ cells in CD4+ and CD8+ cells 56% and 58%, respectively. The erbastatin analog decreases CD69+ cells in CD4+ and CD8+ cells 6% and 21%, respectively, but significantly decreases CD25+ cells in CD4+ cells and CD8+ cells 47% and 55%. To further confirm this effect, tunicamycin was run in a dosage test and was confirmed that it did not affect CD69 (**Figure 4C**) but inhibited other endpoints in a dose-dependent manner including CD25 expression, and the secretion of IFNγ and TNFα.

Using a similar strategy to modify different thresholds in the multi-plate visualization, we also identified the following 3 distinct kinase inhibitors that have no or very moderate inhibition effect on CD25 expression but more inhibitory effect on all other markers including CD69 and IFNγ and TNFα (data not shown: U0126 (MEK1/2 inhibitor), CAY10621 (SPHK1 inhibitor), and bisindolylmaleimide V (S6K inhibitor)). Collectively, these results suggest two potential unique kinase pathways with different spatiotemporal regulation of the early activation markers CD69, and the late activation marker CD25.

3.3.1 Identification of a cluster of MEK1/2 inhibitors with similar activation profiles

Of the 152 kinase inhibitors in the library, there were only 4 MEK1/2 inhibitors. The screening results showed that all 4 compounds broadly inhibit the major relevant markers (CD69 and CD25 expression, and IFNγ and TNFα secretion) after 24-hour T cell activation. The exception was U0126, which had less inhibitory effect on CD25 expression (**Supplemental Figure 2**). **Supplemental Figure 2A** represents the inhibitory effect of MEK1/2 inhibitors on the expression of CD69 and CD25 on both T helper and T cytotoxic cells. **Supplemental Figure 2B** illustrates the decreasing effects on the secretion of the cytokines IFNγ and TNFα. In the subsequent dosage test to confirm the screening results (**Supplement Figure 2C**), 24 IC_{50}s were generated from 4 compounds and 6 endpoints. Two MEK1/2 inhibitors AS703026 and PD0325901 showed strong potency in the inhibition of T cell activation across all 6 major endpoints. All 12 IC_{50}s were less than 0.02 μM. Two MEK1/2 inhibitors, U0126 and PD184161, showed moderate inhibition. A total of 11 IC_{50}s from the latter 2 compounds were greater than 0.3 μM. The exception was PD184161/TNFα with and IC_{50} of 0.072 μM. Although PD184161 had IC_{50}s greater than 10 μM for CD25 expression on T helper and T cytotoxic cells, it does inhibit CD25 expression at the highest tested dose of 10 μM (the dosage curve not shown), similar to the performance in the screening as shown in **Supplement Figure 2A** (see the dark blue columns). High IC_{50}s (greater than the tested highest concentration 10 μM) were due to the lack of the bottom plateau even at the highest dose in the curve fitting.

3.3.2 Identification of 3 distinct kinase inhibitors with similar profiles as a well-known Jak1/2 inhibitor

One commercially valuable compound in the library, ruxolitinib, a myelofibrosis Janus kinase inhibitor with selectivity for subtypes Jak1 and Jak2, is a drug to treat disease. Ruxolitinib was shown as a positive hit in the screening. We used the iQue Forecyt® Profile Map to explore compounds similar to ruxolitinib. In the Profile Map, highlighting the ruxolitinib well triggers the algorithm to place a red tick mark in the slider bars to show the value for each endpoint of the ruxolitinib treatment (**Figure 5A** and **B**). By dragging and minimizing the blue slider bars for each threshold around the red mark (ruxolitinib's position), we identified 3 distinct kinase inhibitors that have profiles similar to ruxolitinib: PKC inhibitor PKC412,

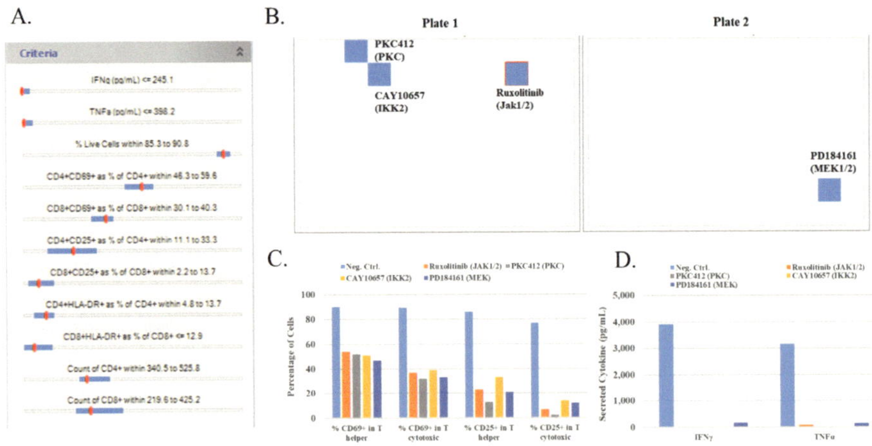

Figure 5.
Identification of a cluster of 3 kinase inhibitors with similar phenotypic signatures as a well-known myelofibrosis drug ruxolitinib (Jak1/2 inhibitor). (A) the 11 criteria that were applied to narrow down the hits that had similar phenotypic signature as ruxolitinib. The B10 well (ruxolitinib) in plate 1 was highlighted in the profile map in iQue Forecyt® software and a red dot corresponding to the B10 wells was highlighted automatically in each threshold Bar by the profile map algorithm. By manually dragging the threshold bar from both the left end and the right end to the red dot (ruxolitinib), compounds with similar profile as ruxolitinib can be identified. Please note, these thresholds can be modified, to get more or fewer hits, according to the user's preference. (B) 3 compounds were identified from 2 screening plates with similar phenotypic signature as ruxolitinib by using the thresholds as seen in the criteria panel (A). (C) Bar graph showing the similar decreasing effect of 3 kinase inhibitors on the cell surface activation markers (CD69 and CD25) in the screening. (D) the bar graph showed the similar strong decreasing effect of 3 kinase inhibitors on the secreted cytokines (IFNγ and TNFα) in the screening.

IKK2 inhibitor CAY10657, and MEK1/2 inhibitor PD184161. It is possible to select a larger or smaller set of compounds with profiles similar to ruxolitinib by choosing a different threshold range for each endpoint. The further quantitative screening results (**Figure 5C** and **D**) suggest these 3 inhibitors, as similar as ruxolitinib, broadly inhibit the T cell activation markers including the expression of CD69 and CD25, and the secretion of cytokine IFNγ and TNFα.

4. Discussion

We developed a novel, immune assay platform that multiplexes cell and bead measurements in the same assay well. The assay analyzes T cell activation from different angles including cell health, time-dependent expression of early activation marker CD69, late activation marker CD25, even later activation marker HLA-DR, and the effector cytokines IFNγ and TNFα. It is also technically possible to multiplex the measurement of other relevant cytokines in T cell activation such as IL-6, IL-10, and IL-17A, depending on biological relevance. Measuring T cell proliferation in the same assay cells involves staining with a cell tracing fluorescent dye prior to assaying. Based on the decrease of fluorescent intensity with each cell division, T cell proliferation can be simultaneously measured.

T cell activation plays a critical role in T cell-mediated tumor cell killing in cancer immunotherapy. This assay could be adapted to measure T cell activation and tumor cell killing simultaneously by barcoding target cells with a cell tracing dye prior to co-culture. A similar assay with CAR-T and tumor cell co-culture was recently reported [22].

Monitoring the condition of T cell activation during the T cell biomanufacturing process is critical to the success of adoptive T cell therapy. As demonstrated in the results (**Figure 1**), this assay may be used for the daily monitoring of T cell activation, and to acquire time-sensitive activation information by checking simultaneously the early or late activation CD markers as well as the major effector cytokine secretion such as IFNγ and TNFα. As a functional assay, it may also be used for profiling neoantigens, vaccines and other drug candidates such as immune checkpoint inhibitors, bi-specific antibodies, as well as inhibitors against inflammation or autoimmune diseases (**Figure 6**).

Using high throughput flow cytometry, this immune assay may be well-suited to the drug screening environment as we demonstrated in the Z' factor characterization. For a proof of concept, we ran a small screening campaign of a chemogenomic kinase library with 152 kinase inhibitors (each with a known target kinase protein). An iQue Forecyt® Profile Map revealed 25 of the total 152 compounds were identified as hits that broadly inhibited the T cell activation parameters, including the early activation marker CD69, the late activation marker CD25, and secreted cytokines IFNγ and TNFα. Furthermore, the first 7 compounds (**Figure 3C**) showed significant inhibition of all parameters (more than 90%, compared with negative control), which suggest an upstream signal pathway simultaneously regulating the expression of all major activation markers such as CD69 and CD25 and the secretion of cytokines IFNγ and TNFα.

However, it might still be an advantage to include both CD69 and CD25 in the same assay for complete insight into the cell activation. As our results suggest, CD69 and CD25 may be decoupled in the downstream signal pathway. This is supported by the finding that 2 compounds from the library screening only inhibit the expression of the late activation marker CD25, but not the early activation marker CD69 (**Figure 4**). This finding is also supported by a similar kinase inhibitor study describing new modulators of T cell receptor signaling and T cell activation [23]. In addition, we found 3 distinct kinase inhibitors that inhibited the early expression marker CD69, but not the late activation marker CD25, which further supports a theory that expression of CD69 and CD25 are regulated differently in downstream

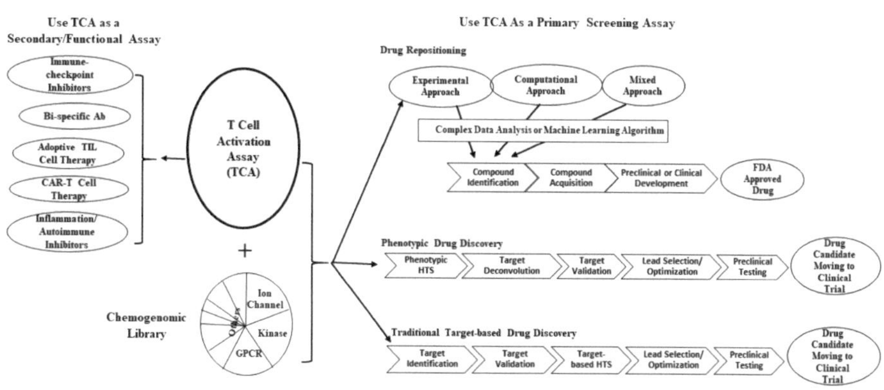

Figure 6.
The potential screening and profiling positions of iQue® human T cell activation kit (TCA assay) in the immune drug discovery workflow. TCA assay may be used as secondary/functional assay to profile the drugs including immune-checkpoint inhibitors, bi-specific antibodies, adoptive TIL cells, CAR-T cells, and inflammation/autoimmune inhibitors. The TCA assay, together with the screening of a chemogenomic library, may be used as primary screening assay for drug repositioning, phenotypic drug discovery and traditional target-based drug discovery.

pathways. In addition, the secretion of the functional cytokines IFNγ and TNFα may not share the same downstream pathway because we identified 2 different compounds (AG17, an EGFR inhibitor and Indirubin-3′-monoxime, a GSK3β inhibitor) that differentially decreased the secretion of one cytokine more drastically than the other (data not shown). Because 24-hour T cell activation was used as a biology model, it was not critical to analyze HLA-DR as an even later activation marker. This marker may be still useful in monitoring T cell activation for a longer term such as 5 to 10 days. The full analysis of different time-sensitive cell surface markers and the secreted cytokines may provide better insight of the precise T cell activation condition.

Of interest were several classes of compounds identified from the library that suggested drug target potential. A cluster of all four MEK1/2 inhibitors from the library showed a similar inhibition profile (**Supplement Figure 2**). In addition, 4 p38MAPK inhibitors, 3 Src kinase inhibitors, and 3 CaMKII inhibitors also showed similar inhibition profiles within each kinase inhibitor family (data not shown). These data suggest that the T cell activation assay, combined with a chemogenomic library screening, has the potential to identify possible drug targets for immune therapy.

In the kinase library screen, a blockbuster kinase inhibitor drug, ruxolitinib (Jak1/2 inhibitor, a myelofibrosis treatment), showed up as a positive hit. By adjusting the hit identification criteria in the iQue Forecyt® Profile Map algorithm, we identified three distinct inhibitors against three different kinase classes. These compounds showed a very similar T cell activation inhibition profile to ruxolitinib. The selection of criteria in the iQue Forecyt® Profile Map algorithm is subjective. It is possible that choosing a different threshold range for each criterion may result in a larger or smaller set of compounds that have inhibition profiles similar to ruxolitinib. In addition, it may be necessary to run in vitro and in vivo validation tests to further confirm the screening results. This small, proof-of-concept screening campaign showed that the multiplexed immune assay, integrated with a sophisticated data analysis algorithms, may help identify compounds or lesser-known existing drugs similar to a well-known drug. This capability may also provide potential new opportunities for kinase drug repositioning, as protein kinases are major oncology drug targets [24].

Aside from drug repositioning, there exists a need to uncover T cell activation biology as it relates to emerging immune-oncology therapies. While immune checkpoint inhibitors such as PD-1 have shown to be effective in mounting an anti-tumor response for both hematologic and solid tumors, there are further mechanistic details related to T cell activation to be learned. For example, a more complete understanding of the interactions between T cell receptors and ligands, upstream of T cell activation, and the modulation of immune checkpoint inhibition, would further progress the immuno-oncology field [25]. Unfortunately, checkpoint inhibitor therapy can result in tumor resistance, due to changes within the tumor cells and/or host immune response [26]. An option to mitigate checkpoint inhibition resistance is to enhance checkpoint inhibition with robust T cell activation via kinase inhibition [27]. Further advances in uncovering T cell activation dynamics as they relate to checkpoint inhibition therapy may include a more complete understanding of how an individual's microbiome might influence cancer treatment. Specifically, the interplay between microbiome diversity, microbiome metabolic signatures, the alteration of T cell activation and the efficacy of checkpoint inhibition therapy has been documented [25].

Both opportunities and challenges exist in phenotypic drug discovery. The small, proof-of-concept screening model described here may be extended to screen other chemogenomic libraries, such as ion channel/GPCR inhibitor, for possible target identification (**Figure 6**), or it may be extended to screen FDA-approved drug libraries for potential drug repositioning purposes. The drug candidates from the screening, particularly against immunological or immuno-oncology targets, can be further profiled by using this immune assay platform or a modified format. With all the characteristics of a functional assay, this assay platform may also be adapted for these applications: neoantigen or vaccine profiling; functional profiling of checkpoint inhibitor and bispecific antibodies in T cell activation and immune cell-mediated tumor cell killing; and daily monitoring T cell activation in the bio-manufacturing of the CAR-T and TIL cells used in adoptive T cell therapy.

5. Conclusions

The ability to readily characterize CD4+ and CD8+ T cell activation state and cytokine secretion is critical for implementing and expanding treatments for cancer, as well as autoimmune and inflammatory conditions. Protein kinase inhibition is an established strategy in oncology treatment, but additional insights are required to expand the portfolio of potential interventions. Key to these efforts is the ability to rapidly and simultaneously monitor cytokines and the temporal expression of T cell activation markers.

This work describes a multiplexed assay screen for protein kinase inhibition to identify compounds that alter T cell activation dynamics. A library of 152 chemogenomic kinase inhibitors was incubated with activated human T cells to determine the expression changes to both early (CD69) and late (CD25) T cell activation markers in conjunction with the cytokine secretion profiles for IFNγ and TNFα from a single assay well. High-throughput flow cytometry screen harnessing integrated, advanced data analytics determined several inhibitors of MEK 1/2 and Jak 1/2 pathways. The existing oncology drug ruxolitinib was identified in the screen and those screen parameters were used to identify 3 additional kinase inhibitors. Importantly, the 3 kinase inhibitor screen hits alter 3 distinct kinase pathways, indicating that this approach is unlikely to show bias for a particular class of kinase activation pathway(s).

6. Future perspectives

Aside from the far-reaching role of T cell activation in cancer treatment, the COVID-19 pandemic has fueled the need for further research of T cell activation dynamics. There is an unmet need to better understand and identify T cell activation related to COVID-19 infection in order to improve COVID-19 treatment [28]. The extent of T cell activation in COVID-19 is associated with either recovery from infection or poor disease prognosis, such as in the cases of severe COVID-19. Interestingly, there is evidence that the enhanced expression of the late stage T cell activation marker HLA-DR is associated with severe COVID-19 [29]. Thus, the ability to perform drug treatment screens, similar to the approach described in this work, and identifying the modulation of T cell activation while simultaneously quantifying cytokine secretion, represents a potentially useful tool for COVID-19 therapeutics as well as for other emerging infectious diseases.

Acknowledgements

We thank all the members of the biology team at Sartorius iQue® for providing comments.

The authors received no financial support for the research, authorship, and/or publication of this article.

Conflict of interest

The authors declare no conflict of interest.

Supplementary material

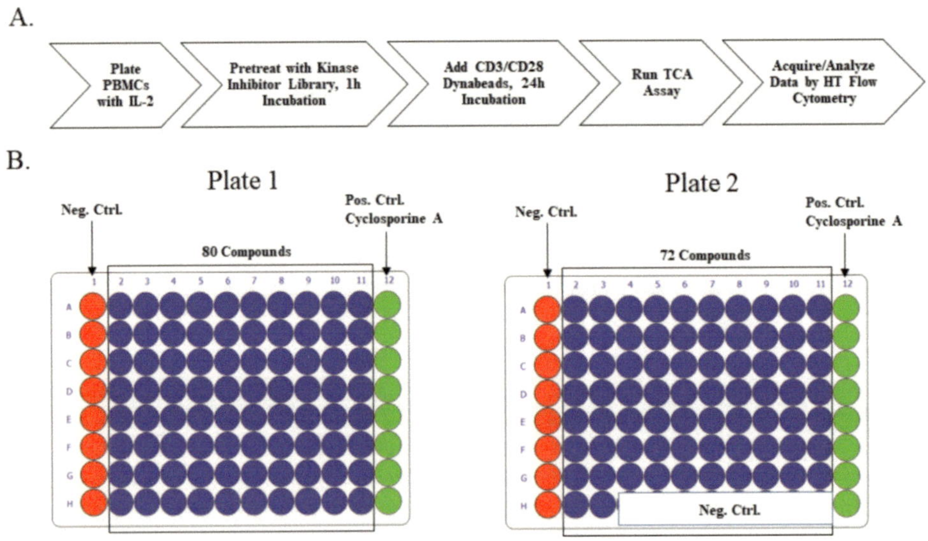

Supplemental Figure 1.
The assay workflow and experimental plate layout for kinase inhibition screening. Supplemental Figure A shows the assay workflow beginning with plating cells, incubating cells with kinase inhibitor, cell activation, assay steps and high-throughput data acquisition. Supplemental Figure B shows the plate map layout showing negative controls in red, sample wells in blue and positive controls in green. The plate map for plate 2 follows the layout of plate one.

A.

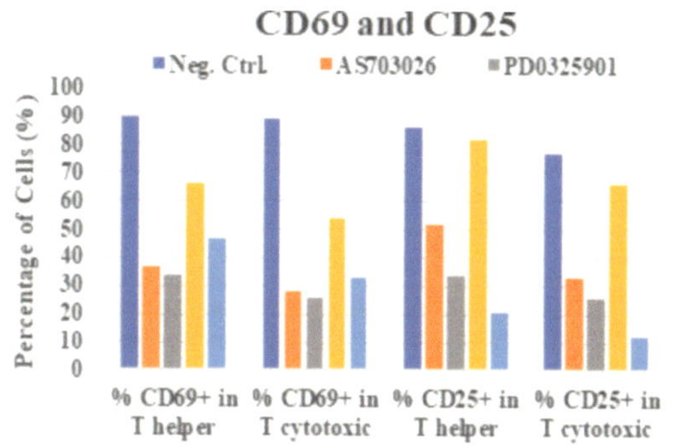

B.

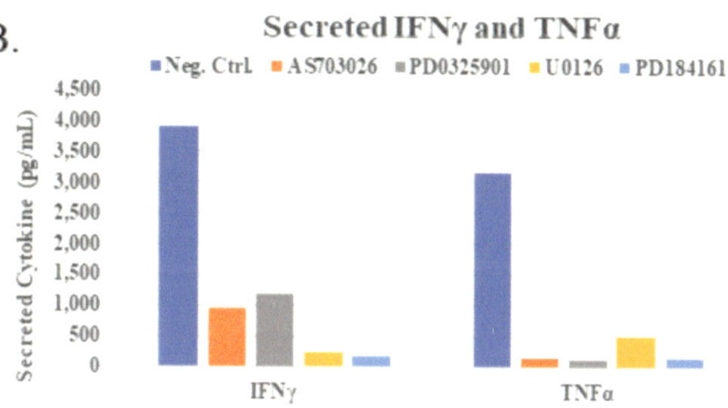

C.

	% CD69+ in T helper	% CD69+ in T cytotoxic	% CD25+ in T helper	% CD25+ in T cytotoxic	IFNγ	TNFα
AS703026	0.008	0.011	0.010	0.019	0.019	0.006
PD0325901	0.012	0.031	0.015	0.017	0.017	0.002
U0126	0.990	3.364	1.237	0.773	0.773	0.314
PD184161	2.560	3.420	>10*	>10*	>10*	0.072

Supplemental Figure 2.
Four MEK1/2 inhibitors that inhibit relevant markers. The screening results showed that all 4 compounds broadly inhibit the major relevant markers (CD69 and CD25 expression, and IFNγ and TNFα secretion) after 24-hour T cell activation. Supplement Figure 2A represents the inhibitory effect of MEK1/2 inhibitors on the expression of CD69 and CD25 on both T helper and T cytotoxic cells. Supplement Figure 2B illustrates the decreasing effects on the secretion of the cytokines IFNγ and TNFα. In the subsequent dosage test to confirm the screening results (Supplement Figure 2C), 24 IC_{50}s were generated from 4 compounds and 6 endpoints.

Appendices and nomenclature

CAR-T	chimeric antigen receptor T cell
TIL	tumor-infiltrating lymphocyte
TCA	assay iQue® Human T Cell Activation Kit assay
ACT	adoptive T cell transfer
MHC	major histocompatibility complex

Author details

Zhaoping Liu*, Andrea Gomez-Donart, Caroline Weldon, Nina Senutovitch and John O'Rourke
iQue® Sartorius, Albuquerque, NM, USA

*Address all correspondence to: zhaoping.liu@Sartorius.com

References

[1] Medicines in Development for Autoimmune Diseases. *Pharmaceutical Research and Manufacturers of America* (PhRMA) 2016.

[2] Tang J, Pearce L, Odonnell-Tormey J, Hubbard-Lucey VM. Trends in the Global Immuno-Oncology Landscape. Nat. Rev. Drug Discov. 2018:17:912–922. DOI: 10.1038/nrd.2018.167

[3] Hosokawa K, Muranski P, Feng X, Townsley DM, Liu B, Knickelbein J, Keyvanfar K, Dumitriu B, Ito S, Kajigaya S, Taylor JG 6th, Kaplan MJ, Nussenblatt RB, Barrett AJ, O'Shea J, Young NS. Memory Stem T Cells in Autoimmune Disease: High Frequency of Circulating CD8+ Memory Stem Cells in Acquired Aplastic Anemia. J Immunol. 2016 Feb 15;196(4):1568–78. DOI: 10.4049/jimmunol.1501739

[4] Schmidt RE, Grimbacher B, Witte T. Autoimmunity and primary immunodeficiency: two sides of the same coin? Nat Rev Rheumatol. 2017 Dec 19;14(1):7–18. DOI: 10.1038/nrrheum.2017.198

[5] Raphael I, Nalawade S, Eagar TN, Forsthuber TG. T cell subsets and their signature cytokines in autoimmune and inflammatory diseases. Cytokine. 2015 Jul;74(1):5–17. DOI: 10.1016/j.cyto.2014.09.011

[6] Sharma P, Allison JP. The future of immune checkpoint therapy. Science. 2015 Apr 3;348(6230):56–61. DOI: 10.1126/science.aaa8172

[7] Thakur A, Huang M, Lum LG. Bispecific antibody based therapeutics: Strengths and challenges. Blood Rev. 2018 Jul;32(4):339–347. DOI: 10.1016/j.blre.2018.02.004

[8] Zacharakis N, Chinnasamy H, Black M, Xu H, Lu YC, Zheng Z, Pasetto A, Langhan M, Shelton T, Prickett T, Gartner J, Jia L, Trebska-McGowan K, Somerville RP, Robbins PF, Rosenberg SA, Goff SL, Feldman SA. Immune recognition of somatic mutations leading to complete durable regression in metastatic breast cancer. Nat Med. 2018 Jun;24(6):724–730. DOI: 10.1038/s41591-018-0040-8

[9] June CH, O'Connor RS, Kawalekar OU, Ghassemi S, Milone MC. CAR T cell immunotherapy for human cancer. Science. 2018 Mar 23;359(6382):1361–1365. DOI: 10.1126/science.aar6711

[10] Almåsbak H, Aarvak T, Vemuri MC. CAR T Cell Therapy: A Game Changer in Cancer Treatment. J Immunol Res. 2016;2016:5474602. DOI: 10.1155/2016/5474602

[11] Antonia SJ, Larkin J, Ascierto PA. Immuno-oncology combinations: a review of clinical experience and future prospects. Clin Cancer Res. 2014 Dec 15;20(24):6258–68. DOI: 10.1158/1078-0432.CCR-14-1457

[12] Navarro MN, Cantrell DA. Serine-threonine kinases in TCR signaling. Nat Immunol. 2014 Sep;15(9):808–14. DOI: 10.1038/ni.2941

[13] Ferguson FM, Gray NS. Kinase inhibitors: the road ahead. Nat Rev Drug Discov. 2018 May;17(5):353–377. DOI: 10.1038/nrd.2018.21

[14] Frémin C, Meloche S. From basic research to clinical development of MEK1/2 inhibitors for cancer therapy. J Hematol Oncol. 2010 Feb 11;3:8. DOI: 10.1186/1756-8722-3-8

[15] Bhullar KS, Lagarón NO, McGowan EM, Parmar I, Jha A, Hubbard BP, Rupasinghe HPV. Kinase-targeted cancer therapies: progress, challenges and future directions. Mol Cancer. 2018 Feb 19;17(1):48. DOI: 10.1186/s12943-018-0804-2

[16] Gross S, Rahal R, Stransky N, Lengauer C, Hoeflich KP. Targeting cancer with kinase inhibitors. J Clin Invest. 2015 May;125(5):1780–9. DOI: 10.1172/JCI76094

[17] Carnevalli LS, Sinclair C, Taylor MA, Gutierrez PM, Langdon S, Coenen-Stass AML, Mooney L, Hughes A, Jarvis L, Staniszewska A, Crafter C, Sidders B, Hardaker E, Hudson K, Barry ST. PI3Kα/δ inhibition promotes anti-tumor immunity through direct enhancement of effector CD8⁺ T-cell activity. J Immunother Cancer. 2018 Dec 27;6(1):158. DOI: 10.1186/s40425-018-0457-0

[18] Abril-Rodriguez, G., Torrejon, D.Y., Liu, W. *et al.* PAK4 inhibition improves PD-1 blockade immunotherapy. *Nat Cancer* **1,** 46–58 (2020). DOI.org/10.1038/s43018-019-0003-0

[19] Ding M, Kaspersson K, Murray D, Bardelle C. High-throughput flow cytometry for drug discovery: principles, applications, and case studies. Drug Discov Today. 2017 Dec; 22(12):1844–1850. DOI: 10.1016/j.drudis.2017.09.005

[20] Sklar LA, Carter MB, Edwards BS. Flow cytometry for drug discovery, receptor pharmacology and high-throughput screening. Curr Opin Pharmacol. 2007 Oct;7(5):527–34. DOI: 10.1016/j.coph.2007.06.006

[21] Yi JS, Cox MA, Zajac AJ. T-cell exhaustion: characteristics, causes and conversion. Immunology. 2010 Apr;129 (4):474–81. DOI: 10.1111/j.1365-2567.2010.03255

[22] Martinez EM, Klebanoff SD, Secrest S, Romain G, Haile ST, Emtage PCR, Gilbert AE. High-Throughput Flow Cytometric Method for the Simultaneous Measurement of CAR-T Cell Characterization and Cytotoxicity against Solid Tumor Cell Lines. SLAS Discov. 2018 Aug;23(7): 603–612. DOI: 10.1177/2472555218768745

[23] Chen EW, Brzostek J, Gascoigne NRJ, Rybakin V. Development of a screening strategy for new modulators of T cell receptor signaling and T cell activation. Sci Rep. 2018 Jul 3;8(1):10046. DOI: 10.1038/s41598-018-28106-5

[24] Knapp S. New opportunities for kinase drug repurposing and target discovery. Br J Cancer. 2018 Apr;118(7): 936–937. DOI: 10.1038/s41416-018-0045-6

[25] Saibil SD, Ohashi PS. Targeting T cell activation in immuno-oncology. Curr Oncol. 2020 Apr;27(Suppl 2): S98-S105. doi: 10.3747/co.27.5285. Epub 2020 Apr 1. PMID: 32368179; PMCID: PMC7193998.

[26] Sharma P, Hu-Lieskovan S, Wargo JA, Ribas A. Primary, Adaptive, and Acquired Resistance to Cancer Immunotherapy. Cell 2017 Feb 9;168 (4):707–723. doi: 10.106/j.cell.2017.01.017. PMID: 28187290; PMCID: PMCID: PMC5391692.

[27] Wang Y, Zhang K, Georgiev P, Wells S, Xu H, Lacey BM, Xu Z, Laskey J, Mcleod R, Methot JL, Bittinger M, Pasternak A, Ranganth S. Pharmacological inhibition of hematopoietic progenitor kinase 1 positively regulates T-cell function. PLoS One. 2020 Dec 3;15(12):e0243145. doi: 10.1371/journal.pone.0243145. PMID: 33270695; PMCID: PMC7714195.

[28] Zheng HY, Xu M, Yang CX, Tian RR, Zhang M, Li JJ, Wang XC, Ding ZL, Li GM, Li XL, He YQ, Dong XQ, Yao YG, Zheng YT. Longitudinal transcriptome analyses show robust T cell immunity during recovery from COVID-19. Signal Transduct Target Ther. 2020 Dec 24;5(1):294. doi: 10.1038/s41392-020-00457-4. PMID: 33361761; PMCID:PMC7758413.

[29] Kuri-Cervantes L, Pampena MB, Meng W, Rosenfeld AM, Ittner CAG, Weisman AR, Agyekum RS, Mathew D, Baxter AE, Vella LA, Kuthuru O, Apostolidis SA, Bershaw L, Dougherty J, Greenplate AR, Pattekar A, Kim J, Han N, Gouma S, Weirick ME, Arevalo CP, Bolton MJ, Goodwin EC, Anderson EM, Hensley SE, Jones TK, Mangalmurti NS, Luning Prak ET, Wherry EJ, Meyer NJ, Betts MR. Comprehensive mapping of immune perturbations associated with severe COVID-19. Sci Immunol. 2020 Jul 15;5 (49):eabd7114. doi: 10.1126/sciimmunol. abd7114. PMID:32669287; PMCID: PMC7402634.